DEATH BY *1,000* PAPER CUTS

*How to Achieve a Healthier You
for a Healthier World*

Anton Chumak Andryakov

DEATH BY 1,000 PAPER CUTS: HOW TO ACHIEVE A HEALTHIER YOU FOR A HEALTHIER WORLD

1405 SW 6th Avenue • Ocala, Florida 34471 • Phone 352-622-1825 • Fax 352-622-1875
Website: www.atlantic-pub.com • Email: sales@atlantic-pub.com
SAN Number: 268-1250

Library of Congress Cataloging-in-Publication Data

Names: Chumak Andryakov, Anton, 1986- author.
Title: Death by 1,000 papercuts : how to achieve a healthier you for a healthier world / Anton Andryakov.
Description: Ocala, Florida : Atlantic Publishing Group, Inc., [2019] | Summary: "Thousands of small, re-peated mistakes are detrimental to our personal health as well as the health of society in general. To reverse the downward course of our health, we must make changes one step at a time"— Provided by publisher.
Identifiers: LCCN 2019048646 (print) | LCCN 2019048647 (ebook) | ISBN 9781620237007 (paperback) | ISBN 9781620237014 (ebook)
Subjects: LCSH: Self-care, Health—Popular works. | Health—Popular works. | Mind and body—Popular works. | Nutrition—Popular works.
Classification: LCC RA776.95 .A533 2019 (print) | LCC RA776.95 (ebook) | DDC 613—dc23
LC record available at https://lccn.loc.gov/2019048646
LC ebook record available at https://lccn.loc.gov/2019048647

Printed in the United States

PROJECT MANAGER: Katie Cline
INTERIOR LAYOUT AND JACKET DESIGN: Nicole Sturk

TABLE OF CONTENTS

INTRODUCTION

We usually do not cause damage to our lives through one gaping wound that we can quickly feel and identify. Instead, it is a very gradual process where we do not become aware of the damage until it is too late. It is a painful thought, but I want you to imagine this process as 1,000 tiny paper cuts that cause your body to bleed out ever so slowly. On its own, a paper cut is no big deal. When the same process recurs daily in many different but related areas, we can start causing a massive problem. Now when that process keeps occurring for years, we can face things like the loss of a limb, as in the case of diabetes, or something way more severe, including death.

Because this process is so gradual and the daily changes are incredibly subtle, we do not see the impact on our lives. We change so slightly every day that it seems that it is not really occurring. Over time, however, those changes bring us to a place where we no longer recognize ourselves physically, mentally, spiritually, and financially. In life, we need contrast to make judgments and assessments. When the changes are so small, we often do not see the necessary contrast until it is too late. For example, when you slowly gain weight, you may not notice it until you finally step on a scale after not doing so for a while. You may not have been motivated to change your physique before, but the sharp contrast of the weight change makes you realize how much you gained. Suddenly, your motivation increases. If you do not remember what you felt like at your old weight, that motivation may not kick in as much because you have accepted your current reality as permanent. When the change is slow and gradual, it takes us a long time to notice the need to go back to our old selves. If that time is far away and we have forgotten what that good feeling is like, we are going to struggle with the motivation to get there. We have a harder time finding the motivation to return to that optimal state that we all should strive for. How could we want to work for something if we no longer can see its value?

There is a difference between living, surviving, and thriving. This book focuses on the health aspect of thriving. I will cover an abundance of concepts, but the intention is not to give you an in-depth knowledge of each one. The intent is to show you how doing these things wrong every day are like paper cuts each time that can lead to a life where you are just surviving. My desired outcome for you is not to become an expert. I want you to identify areas where you need to grow. Most importantly, I want to empower you to ask better health-related questions. This book will give you the ability to see the whole forest from 30,000 ft. rather than the view from walking in the middle.

I dedicate the book to my father. He has been gone for over 25 years now and was taken way too soon from this earth. He made thousands of tiny paper cuts throughout his life that ended up taking him out of this world at a very early age of 45. Seeing him on his death bed, I knew that, had he had this knowledge and the proper support, he could have been around for 40 more years. This book is a wake-up call for a disconnected society that has no care for its future health. We no longer worry about our health as our grandparents did. You simply do not hear talk of disease aversion and late-onset health issues like you would 30-50 years ago. You live in willful ignorance, and you often use the word "just" as a reason why you knowingly do something wrong for your mental, spiritual, or physical health.

You cannot do what you do now without consequences, and the ones I talk about do not show up until 10-15 years down the road.

Some, of course, occur more quickly than that. The issue is that you do not make the connection between the problem and the original action, so you continue those detrimental steps. If you picked up this book because you want to lose weight, that is great, but there are many more significant benefits. This book will help you play with your grandkids, enjoy retirement, and live a life of fulfillment. That all comes from eating well, moving more, and managing the internal aspects of your health, like your brain and blood chemistry. You will uncover all the mistakes so you either avoid them or recognize when you are making them so you can course correct.

Have you ever heard of Earth Overshoot Day? For most, this day is unknown. But for people who are very passionate about sustainability, this day is a big deal. Earth Overshoot Day marks the day that humans have used up the resources on this planet for the year. The remainder of the year is the overshoot, or the amount we are going into debt with the planet. I am sure I do not need to explain how using up our yearly resources before August is not a sustainable way of living. But I want to use this concept and apply it to a bigger problem that exists in our society.

Similar to how Mother Earth has limited resources, our mind, body, and spirit are the same way. We only have so many hours in the day for our system to do the work, rest, and then be able to repeat the process. We only have so many nutrients we can put in our body to help it function as designed and can only filter out so many bad things we put inside of us. There are only so many things our mind can focus on before it gets burned out. All of this makes sense, but we are not living this way. Since I came to the United States in 1999, each year I have seen more and more overload on our society and the human beings within it. That overload comes from stress and mistreating our mind, body, and spirit by eating poorly, not exercising regularly, and not paying attention to our internal blood and brain chemistry.

I do not know about you, but this scares me to my core. Why? It has to do with how long it took our society to become more conscious of the environmental problems created by living in an unsustainable way. I consider the hippies, who started to push the green movement, for the creation of this awareness. However, it was not until 2007 that Earth Overshoot Days began to occur at later dates in the year. So, this means that it took our society somewhere around 45 measuring occurrence of Earth Overshoot Days before the slowdown began.

When applying the same logic to our health, it is scary to consider that the change will not happen until the mid-2040s. Can you imagine the state of our communities if humans keep operating like we are for the next 25 years? Can we not repeat the mistakes of the past and create a more significant movement for human sustainability and health, be it in everyday life or in our work? I think as many people are on board with making the earth greener as they were in the early '60s. Yet we must consider, are we willing to make the necessary sacrifice to preserve our bodies and levels of happiness?

This book is broken up into many "paper cuts" that we make on a regular basis. It is organized into four categories of health: mindset, internal health, nourishment, and movement. All four components are vital to having a thriving, health focused life.

PART 1

Mindset

CHAPTER 1

Giving 100% Away Paper Cut

It was 5:30 a.m. when I was woken up from some commotion in our apartment. There were many more people there than usual, as my grandmother and grandfather were with us and awaiting the inevitable that finally came that morning. The setting was Russia in 1995, and we lived in a one-bedroom apartment that had a large balcony, which became my bedroom. As I made my way through the living space, I walked into the common area. My mom and my grandma ran up to me in tears, and instantly I knew something was gravely wrong. They brought me into the living room where my parents had lived for the eight years I had been alive. For the last two years, the living room had been getting harder and harder to spend time in. It had become the hospital room for my father, who was fighting lymphoma.

I looked over at my father's bed and saw a sheet covering his entire body; my mom told me that my father had passed away that morning. It was not a surprise to the family. It had been a very long and hard battle, where my father had withered away slowly and almost nothing but skin and bones remained. Since I was eight at the time, I did not have a full comprehension of what was happening. I was quickly taken to my grandmother's house so as not to be around as my family prepared to bury my father. The moment I just described is the second most vivid memory of my childhood.

My most vivid memory happened a few days later. This memory would later lead to an understanding that would set the trajectory for my health-driven mission and bring me to write this book. We lived in a large apartment building that would make you think of the buildings that are in the projects in the U.S. My father was a big deal in our city before the USSR fell apart; he was the beloved mayor that moved mountains for his people. Although it had been four years since he was in that role, my family was preparing for many people to come and pay their respects. However, nobody anticipated the size of the crowd creating standing room only in the courtyard, where his casket was on display. I was not allowed to go to the cemetery, but when I was leaving to go to my grandma's house, I saw a two mile long line of people walking to pay their respects. Even if they had not met him face to face before, the man they came to honor had meant that much to them.

Why am I telling you about this in a health-oriented book? The reason is simple. When I became a health and wellness professional, I did it with a desire to prevent people from following my father's path. When I got out of the Marine Corps, I thought about this vivid memory, and it led me to a way of thinking. My father was an amazing man, and he gave 100 percent of himself to his purpose and his people every day. What if he had just kept 10 percent of himself for himself? How much longer could he have been on this planet, serving his purpose? How many more lives could he have impacted? Everyone who knew my father would agree that not just he, but all of us would have benefited much more. We would have been so happy having him around at a 90 percent capacity for the rest of the 30-40 years that he should have lived. The logic makes sense, but we do not act on this logic in our society. We are not logical creatures by nature. It may seem like a no-brainer, but our emotional side takes over and causes things to go in another direction.

I see this happening often with parents, entrepreneurs, leaders, and many other people with a great purpose on their minds. They give away 100 percent of their capacity to bring this purpose into fruition not realizing that each day, from many repeated paper cuts, their potential to give diminishes. It becomes a process of diminishing returns. As they try to work harder and do more, they get less accomplished. Do any of you ever feel like you are in this same cycle?

To explain what occurs in these situations, I will use a gas tank analogy. When you embarked on the mission of bringing your purpose to life, you were your most energetic, passionate, driven, and optimized self. You had a five gallon gas tank that allowed you to create an impressive impact. Like my father, you started to give 100 percent of that gas tank away daily to serve the purpose you were after. That is amazing, and the world is better for it. But this behavior is not sustainable because, over time, the capacity to give shrinks. After years, you continue to give 100 percent of your gas toward this purpose, but the problem becomes that, due to not nurturing yourself, you now only have a one gallon gas tank. Once again, when we look at this logically, it makes perfect sense. So why do we not do the right thing?

It is because our emotions often take over, and before we can make logical assessments, they end up clouding our judgment. We begin to measure our impact based on the feeling of effort we are putting in rather than the logical measurement of the actual outcome. We feel an emotional guilt that we must keep giving more while not realizing, logically, that our impact is greatly reduced as we continue this practice. If you keep 10 percent of yourself for yourself, you will be able to give 90 percent of that five gallon gas tank for as long as you are around. The other area that you are making a mistake in, is that you are comparing apples to oranges. By that I mean you examine your outcomes and see that you may still be producing the same amount of them as you were with a five gallon tank all these years later. This makes you think that you have not diminished your potential. The problem is that we expect a much higher level of output because we have grown over the years and have more tools and knowledge that we can apply to deliver results. Hence, if the knowledge and experience grew, we should be creating a much higher output. But it does not happen, or at least to the degree expected, because the gas tank has shrunk. We are lost in the rat race, oblivious to the logic right in front of our noses.

This is one of many reasons why the #10PercentFITTER method was created. The entire contents of this book are part of this method that I developed. It is also my gift to the world in honor of my father. By the time this book is published, I will have released the entire method to the world for free. It is my way of trying to raise world health by at least 10 percent through creating an open source health knowledge platform. You can go to **www.prospectiveforce.com/10percentfitter** to gain access to all the knowledge for free.

This book will cover many great options as to what you can do to fill that 10 percent. You want to ensure you are always running on not just a full tank, but one that has its capacity for output growing with time. You do not need to do all the things that I cover in this book, nor do you need to stop doing all the things that hurt you. If you stop doing some and start doing others, you will see the massive positive impact and get closer to becoming your optimized self. In turn, you will create points of contrast that will motivate you to seek further improvement over time until you reach your peak potential in body and mind.

This book intentionally covers a vast amount of information with shallow depth. There are many excellent books and resources you can use to get more in-depth knowledge. My goal is to help you to see the bigger picture and learn to ask better questions when you need to go deeper. Too often, we start with details and do not see how to connect the dots in all things we are working on in life. I do not want you to do that so you can become more self-sustained with your health. When you gain enough knowledge, your motivation improves as it makes you feel as if you are mastering something. I will talk about intrinsic motivation in a later chapter, but it is vital to make changes that you will stick with for a lifetime, instead of making surface level changes that lead to your reverting back to the original behaviors.

Accepting the fundamental mindset of keeping 10 percent of yourself for yourself is the first step to improving your health and maximizing your performance. Before you act, you need to have the right framework of thoughts and beliefs, and this is at the foundation of all of it.

CHAPTER 2

Jump Before You Are Ready
Paper Cut

It is so exciting to commit to a personal change, especially when it involves improving your health. You see the destination you are heading toward, and you are excited to get to that point B on your journey. Hope fills your mind and heart, and you go 100 percent all-in. There is just one problem. Whenever you navigate using a map or a GPS app to get to your destination, you must know your point of origin. Understanding and evaluating the starting point will ensure that the plan you have created fits the situation you are facing. This statement rings even more accurate when it comes to your health because typically you are in a hole that you dug from years of bad choices. You must consider your four resources for success whenever you embark on any journey: your time, your mindset, your support, and of course, your budget. The four resources are not in any particular order of importance, as each one of them is just as vital as the other. I will break down each one and why they are essential. This knowledge will help you avoid making the paper cut of not paying attention to the starting point on your health journey.

Most people think money is the most limiting resource they have. I strongly disagree with that perspective. When I worked in the corporate world, the sales I made were in a face-to-face environment, at a physical location. There was a concept I would use to illustrate to my clients that money was not the reason they were not willing to commit to the program. I would tell a person that I have a body shop downstairs. For $20,000 they could pick out any body they wanted, and we would switch the heads, and they could have it. I would ask if they would max out every credit card to make that happen. The answer was almost always yes, even though they objected to the price at first. Why does this phenomenon occur? People do not assess themselves thoroughly. When they say no due to budgetary constraints, many are saying that the result they foresee getting from the product or service is not worth the investment. Often it has nothing to do with the product or the service, but everything to do with the person's lack of belief in themselves to stay committed. It is this fear of failure that is being hidden by a concern for money.

To start, let's investigate money and, besides the obvious, why it is so important to consider this resource before embarking on your health journey. What kinds of things are needed that may require money? As our society becomes more advanced, we get additional options on how to invest our budgets with so many different health choices. We look at celebrities that are very fit and envy them, comparing our life to theirs. This comparison is not fair as it compares apples to oranges. They have enough money to afford a personal chef, a trainer five days a week, a nutrition coach to guide their every step, and the best supplements and lab tests that exist. Your financial situation may not allow for this. This means that you need to have a different set of expectations. The celebrities may be able to get in the best shape of their life in three months, but it may take you one full year to get there. The more money you have, the more challenges to complete things by yourself fall to the side. Does it mean that, without money, it is impossible? No, it just means that the other three resources will have to be depleted more to compensate. You may have to learn nutrition and give up time. You may have to shift your mindset to celebrate smaller wins, knowing you are running a marathon and not a sprint. You may have to enlist support, that could have gone elsewhere, to help you in areas for which you do not have the money. All these considerations are incredibly important to plot an accurate journey for your health changes.

Personally, time is the resource I cherish and maximize the most. Why? I can buy support, I can always get more money, and I can get help with my psychology. But no matter what I do, I cannot get more time. When I was 18 years old and finishing out my senior year of high school, I had all the time in the world. I did not have a job, a partner, kids, or a house I had to maintain. I was in the best shape of my life. I had 100 percent to give to my health. Now I am well into my 30s with a wife, three kids, three dogs, two companies, and plenty of other responsibilities. Giving 100 percent of myself to anything is impossible, even when it is something as important as my health. This is why I have created my #10PercentFITTER Method to help those that are in a similar situation. You must be reasonable with the time you have to give to your health and have the right plan that fits that. Going for the all-or-nothing approach, that so many succumb to after spending too much time on social media, will not serve you.

People will often consider budget and time when starting their journey, but overlook psychology and support. When I speak of psychology, I mean two things. First, your readiness to change, and second, your mindset. We often do not consider how ready we are to create change in our lives. To help, I want to present the six stages that you could be in, when considering implementing a change. First comes the precontemplation stage. This stage is where you are looking at what other people are doing, but you do not identify that what you are observing is an actual problem in your life. The contemplation stage is when you are still dragging your feet, but you now see that you are part of the problem. As you begin to face the challenge and own it, you enter the preparation stage. You are doing some test runs to practice how you could tackle this issue. Then comes the action stage, where you begin to implement the plan and the tools needed to create the desired change. After that, you face the maintenance stage, which people often overlook. The focus here is to ensure that the changes already made become foundational before moving on to the next revisions. Last, but most certainly not least, is the relapse stage. This stage is where you will go back to your old ways, and the focus is to get back on track as fast as possible. Also, you will want to create a plan that, over time, makes the relapses further and further apart. I cannot count on my hands and feet how many potential clients I said no to, because I saw that they were only at the precontemplation stage. They needed to be more ready to get the return on their desired investment. I always believe that not every sale is a good sale and understanding the person's readiness for change is a significant determining factor in that.

Now that you are ready and have worked up to action stage, the next vital thing to consider is your mindset. In this area, you must set yourself in the right direction of thinking by answering these questions the right way: Why are you making this change? Who is this going to impact, and is it for you or to appease someone else? What will life be like if you do not make this change? What can life be like if you do? How will you avoid the all-or-nothing approach? How will you celebrate small wins along the way, to create a winning momentum? How will you stand up to naysayers that do not believe in you? How will you be prepared to face potential obstacles? How are you going to make sure to make small, yet mighty, changes? When you learn to answer these questions the right way, it means that you have learned to control your internal narrative, often a massive roadblock to people's success.

When considering your resources for success, support cannot be missed. We need assistance, and if we do not have it around us at that moment, we may need to use some of the other resources to gain it. I have seen many divorces happen because one spouse made health changes and the other did not. If they had been a support system for each other from the start, chances are, they would still be happily married. It is always best to get your partner on board. When that is not possible, you still need to consider them when making the changes. We can have people as support, but some can become the opposite: the ball and chain we drag around daily. There will come a time when you may need to change relationships or terminate friendships. This is a natural life cycle as people grow apart when they change careers and environments. Similarly, people can grow apart when their health status changes. Because when we change health, we do not just change our appearance; we change our thinking, energy, drive, and so many other pivotal life factors. You need people in your corner, but you also need to get rid of the ones that may hold you back. That is okay because all of this is to be selfishly selfless. By putting your health first, you will be that much more impactful in other areas of your life. That way, you will help others in the process.

CHAPTER 3

Perpetual Dieting Paper Cut

You are what you eat. Have you heard that statement before? Our digestion and ability to absorb food and nutrients has a lot to do with that statement. It is not always accurate, but for now, let's run with that common belief. Nutrition has been part of health conversations for longer than we have had formal civilizations. For thousands of years, eating roots and extracts has been a go-to form of medicine. With that said, anything that is good, can also be bad. The way that most of us are eating these days is damaging to our body. In this chapter, we will examine the critical components of a healthy diet as well as dive into some present options for nutritional guidance. Nutrition is one of the most frequent causes of the life paper cuts that hurt us, and we will cover a lot of it in this book. You will learn that nutrition connects to areas of your life you may not have expected. This connection is essential to shifting your relationship with food into a positive one.

Throughout my 10 plus years of coaching on nutrition, I have taken many approaches with over 300 clients. I have employed fad diets and behavior modification techniques to help clients lose or gain weight, ultimately optimizing their bodies. If you were to buy a Ferrari, would you skip regular oil changes or put the cheapest gas into it? No, you would do all the maintenance and give it the best fuel possible. Yet we do not treat our body, which is more precious than a Ferrari, in the same way. Why is that? We can buy a new Ferrari, but we are not able to buy a new body. Our bodies are meant to be the most amazing pieces of machinery in the world, but they require proper maintenance and the right fuel to operate that way. You are built for survival, so you can withstand a lot of the damage you inflict via improper nutrition. But we must remember that we do not want to survive this life. We want to thrive in life, and what we put in our mouth has more to do with it than anything else.

With so much contradicting information out there, people have become increasingly lost in what is the right or wrong nutritional choice. What we believed for many years as absolute truth can be refuted a few years from now. We always have to wear a hat of caution when making nutritional choices, which is why I lean on simplicity.

One of the biggest things I can teach you that has helped all my clients is to start small, think big, and move fast to get to your desired goals. The first piece of advice is very crucial. You must start small with a singular habit. You understand that you should not walk into the gym on day one and throw 300 lbs. over your head. For some reason, when it comes to nutrition, you tend not to apply this same principle. You like to create this massive plan that may include all or some of the following: meal plans, a macronutrient break down, tracking and measuring food, eating six meals a day, only eating 50 grams of carbs a day, and many others. This approach requires too much change for our minds to make a permanent transition, and it ends up being a short-lived diet that creates more problems down the road. Why is that? The reason is that our body cannot take on too much change at once. We must focus on one change at a time because, statistically speaking, when making just one change, we have an 80 percent success rate according to precisionnutrition. com. When we increase to two changes, that success rate drops to 35 percent, and when we do three changes or more at once, the success rate drops below 10 percent.

Your goal should be the same as the goal that I have for all my clients: achieve results today, maintain them a year from now, and ensure it does not hinder your health 15 years from now. There are many gimmicky diets out there that can give you results today. The problem is that they cannot be maintained long term or, even worse, they can hurt your health many years down the road. This is why I am against the HCG diet because it wrecks bodies, especially women's hormones. After HCG disruption, it is nearly impossible to fix the metabolism and get back on a healthy track. According to the Mayo Clinic, FDA has made a caution for people to steer clear of diet products containing HCG, yet it is still a booming business.

Another thing to steer clear from is using diet pills. Many of them are packed with caffeine to elicit a thermogenic effect and increase metabolism. This increase may be beneficial for caloric burn, but it can hurt other areas of the body, like your adrenal glands that regulate stress. These pills may give you results today, and maybe you can maintain them a year from now. But most likely they will start a chain of events that will lead to poor health 15 years from now, specifically in the form of your adrenal glands not functioning correctly. This disfunction can cause all sorts of issues, including raising your risk for cancer and other stress-related ailments.

I am not here to say that all diets are wrong, but I do not believe in the process unless it is for a medical need. Later, I will go over some diets that I have used with clients, while also teaching them correct nutritional habits. Those habits, with time, replace the need for dieting. And why do diets sound so enticing to us? It is the quick fix appeal that marketers use to make us believe they are the perfect solution. They appeal to our emotional side, and then logic goes out the window and we choose to go on this diet. It is similar to how people make millions by selling people get rich quick schemes. Logic tells us that if we are to build something great and sustainable, like a healthy nutritional intake, it will take time. The problem is that our emotions push us toward a solution that promises to solve all our issues by tomorrow.

My biggest problem with dieting is that people often grasp a portion of the concept and start running 100 miles per hour trying to implement it. They usually do not understand that they need to custom-tailor the large plan to their lifestyle, which is of utmost importance for success. This lack of understanding, in turn, leads to inevitable failure. Then we get more emotional scarring that creates more of a problem in our relationship with food. When we step away from emotion and break down dieting on a logical basis, we see the reality.

I want you to think about a few chronic dieters that you know in your life. Chances are, if they fall into the statistical majority, you have witnessed their weight yo-yo over the last 10-15 years. Chances are, if they have been dieting this long, they have steadily gained weight from their initial starting point. When we perpetually diet it is a constant up and down effect. There are many peaks and there are many valleys, but over time, both the peaks and the valleys end up higher than at the start of dieting beliefs. Why does that happen? Because diets are like a bandage to the problem; they do not solve the root of the problem and help to mask the symptoms. The source of the problem is that our metabolism is not functioning correctly due to many possible disruptors. I will dive into this in a later chapter, discussing how to identify where the issue truly lies and how to fix it so that your weight, energy, and performance are improved permanently. The reason diets are one of the biggest and most common paper cuts is the common yet false understanding that we are doing something good for our bodies.

As you learn the many application tools in this book, remember that you are on a plan that looks more like a marathon instead of a short burst sprint. This mindset means that you implement one change at a time until it becomes a habit, and then you move on to the next one once you have established consistency. I know you are tired of living the way you are right now but trying to change it overnight will not be productive. Just think, if you had been making one change at a time rather than dieting for however long you have been trying to improve your health, how far could you be by now? Make sure you stop this mistake so a year from now you can be further along than you ever dreamed. These seemingly small mistakes are actually many of the paper cuts that lead our body into a metabolic mess that can take up to a year of supervised coaching to correct. Countless people never get there because of the long term need for consistency.

Start small, think big, move fast!

CHAPTER 4

Goal Setting Paper Cut

Discussion around goal setting has become one of the most common topics in self-development, and even in business circles. There is so much pressure to dream big and go for it. Many people teach you the action of setting goals but do not consider the psychology and the custom-tailored need in the application. It is as if we are all on the same journey, with the same starting point and desired destination. We know that's not the case and need to see that this in itself is a considerable paper cut. We end up following a journey that is not for us, and then we beat ourselves up when we are not successful. This misalignment is a big problem, and we need to address it as our subconscious is being hurt by it daily. Most of our choices and actions are not conscious decisions but are made automatically to simplify our brain's operation. When we do not follow a goal-setting process and go after things too quickly, we prime our subconscious for self-doubt. This doubt minimizes the potential we hold within us.

This understanding rings true in any area of life, but it is extremely common in health. Let me unpack this problem a bit here in this chapter. I want you to think about your business or something that you have mastered. If I came to you and said we have a goal of no longer making mistakes at work, would that be realistic? Or if I came to you and said that by next week, we are going to grow your top-line revenue by 200 percent, does that seem like a goal that you would set? No, because you know all the smaller steps that would have to occur for that to happen, even if it was possible. You have gone through this experience and understand that this goal would not be just a point A to point B, but would be more like a point A to point Z. Every letter represents a step in the process. However, when we want to shift our own behavior, we do not apply this concept.

When it comes to health, we tend to forget all the steps. Right now, you may be eating a ton of junk food and skipping regular meals. It is possible that you have a deficiency of nutritional knowledge. What makes you think you can wake up tomorrow and follow this perfect diet a 24-year-old guy with abs sold you on Instagram? We keep failing and spending more money on gimmicks, never realizing that what we see as A to B is A to Z. This repeated failure makes us give up eventually, and we keep looking for easy fixes that lead to nowhere, if not sending us backwards.

So how do you set health goals that will work for you? How do you do that all while achieving results tomorrow, maintaining them a year from now, and not negatively impacting your health 15 years down the road? Well, before you plot a path of where you are going, you need to become very aware of where you currently are. We often overestimate the quality of our nutritional intake and our ability to make changes.

For example, when you are trying to get better with nutrition, take a look at your current situation by starting a food diary. Log every time you eat and what you eat. If you want to go deeper, I suggest logging what you feel as well. You must understand that it is not just the choices you make with food, it is where those decisions might be coming from, emotionally and environmentally. I promise you that you will uncover some patterns that need to be changed and from there, tackle them one at a time. Remember your health correction journey is not a sprint; it is a long-distance marathon and requires patience and persistence. Your health did not get into this hole overnight, and you cannot climb out that fast either.

Now that you have completed your self-assessment and identified your opportunities, it is time to move on to the goal setting process. You want to utilize the acronym S.M.A.R.T. when setting those goals, and it breaks down to mean Specific, Measurable, Attractive, Realistic, and Timely. Many people will focus on Specific, Measurable and Timely components being the most important. I like to look at the Realistic one the most. I am sure you have heard many people say that when you set your goals, you should shoot for the moon because even if you miss and don't get there, you will end up amongst the stars. This kind of stuff is great for motivational speeches and social media posts, but when it comes to behavior change, it is a massive paper cut that many people do not even notice. Now I am not saying you should not dream big, but it is more important to focus on the next step and celebrate each achievement as much as you would reaching your goal.

The first goal you must set is something that can be very short-term and is not based on an outcome, but on merely taking action. Here, you should not say I want to lose x number of pounds. Instead, say I want to improve my blood sugar regulation, but it has to start with correcting my current behavior. If before you were not eating more than three meals and a couple of snacks a day, your short-term behavior goal could be to follow that meal plan for five days. Weekends can be tough and I want to create a win for you so starting with the weekdays and nailing that down could be a great place to begin.

Now, you are achieving your first goal for a few weeks in a row and are starting to believe in yourself. You see the positive effects of your actions in the way you feel, and you may be ready for a long-term behavior goal that builds on your success. An example of this could be doing a 30-day elimination of food that may be against your goals. I had a client that came to me because she was struggling with getting leaner. She was already very fit and wanted a six-pack. I knew right away there were bigger things at play than just helping her lose that last few percent of her body fat, but being a coach meant I had to meet her where she was. She ate clean, and her macronutrients were always where they should be, yet she could no longer move the needle with her fat reduction. She would train as hard as she could but was not seeing results on her stomach. After doing some assessments with her, I uncovered that it was due to stress. She did not have a lot of mental stress, and her job was very easy for her, so she could not understand when I told her that her body was stressed out. Frustrated and eventually breaking down in tears, she told me some information about her digestive symptoms that made me realize that her stress was coming from there. She was a long-distance performance athlete, and through the constant rigor of her sport, she was hurting her digestion. The fix was a lot simpler than you might think. We did an elimination diet and figured out that any time she had yeast, she would experience a little bloating and post-meal fatigue. This indicated to me that yeast had to be avoided. I will cover what to do to fix digestion later, but first we had to make a behavior goal for her. I had her stop focusing on the final goal of losing body fat in her stomach and shift her mindset toward healing her gut. I had her commit to a 30-day elimination plan where she could eat anything she wanted, but it could not have any baker's yeast as that was the type of yeast that had the strongest negative response. It was fun because she had a feeling of winning again, which she could not get from outcome-based goals. You know how vital that winning momentum is when trying to accomplish things. Through that, we started to see a change again, and we shifted her goals to a higher level goal.

The next level is the most common type of goal, the outcome-based goal. Whether it is losing a certain amount of weight, correcting a health problem like type 2 diabetes, or achieving a certain look, these goals focus on the actual end of the journey. My advice to you here is to ensure that this goal is not too large so you are not skipping steps, thinking it is an A to B type of goal, where in reality, it is an A to Z. Once again, using the mentality of starting small, thinking big, moving fast is the best way to go about these goals. It will continue that winning momentum that will keep you on track with your motivation. The outcome-based goals are the ones that use the S.M.A.R.T. principle the most. They also require a bit more planning and will actually include many behavior-based goals within the process to the desired destination. This type of goal is where most people stop even though two more levels remain.

Remember that when you are trying to achieve any goal, you are trying to influence yourself positively. The rules do not change here, and we must remember that when we try to influence others or ourselves. There are three paths to get there: ethos, logos, and pathos are derived from old philosophical writing. They mean that to influence a decision, we can use ethos, which is ethical ground, logos, which is logical persuasion, and pathos, which is an emotional appeal. Now ask yourself, when you make most of your decisions, how do you make them? If you are like the majority of the world, chances are the way you feel about something has a lot to do with your ability to execute it to fruition. Yet, we have not focused much on that aspect with the three levels of goals.

Yes, we will always connect a "why" to any goal that we do, but I am talking about something that sets your soul on fire with passion. This brings me to the fourth goal in the goal progression cycle: the passion goal. This is a long-term goal, but it still has an end to it and is something that we are extremely passionate to accomplish. This one takes time to identify, and many components must be present. Passion goals are not goals I recommend setting in a quick thinking session. For this goal, I encourage you to spend a day by yourself in nature, and figure out what it is you are enthusiastic about and how you want to use that passion to drive you to be better. Simple examples could be to do a competition of some sort like a marathon, a bodybuilding contest, or a survival race. More complex goals could be like my own goal to make a difference in the way people live their lives in order to create a more humanly sustainable society. Another example could be someone wanting their kids to become the best versions of themselves and get into an Ivy League school.

There are so many different goals that can be set at this level, and they are super individual, as they depend on a person's passion. If this is something you cannot pinpoint, it means you have some identity searching to do, and that is a whole other conversation. I also work with people on identifying their passions, and it is one of the hardest yet most beneficial things you will ever do for yourself. The reason this goal comes later is because it takes the mastery and the winning momentum of the first three to be able to reach for this long-term one. Even though you may have a huge passion for something, it does not mean that you can maintain the journey without breaking it up into smaller components and making yourself feel like you are making progress and doing the right thing.

So far, every goal we have discussed has an end. There is one big problem around goals that have an end: the concept of "close enough" starts to creep in. I will discuss how motivation works later but know that our body is continually evaluating the work that we have to do and the outcome that work brings. The last 5 to 10 percent of our results are the hardest to achieve sometimes. I learned this from many clients that set out to lose weight. They may want to lose 40 lbs. but often stop around 30 to 35 lbs. because the last five pounds are much harder than the initial five. This seemingly insignificant failure often causes people to fall off their journey and discontinue the behaviors that got them close in the first place.

I learned this through one of my clients a few years back. He was a pilot, and he got in terrible shape from all the stress and lack of structure in his life due to his intense schedule. He was about 35 percent body fat when he came to me for help. We created a plan that was diet and cardio focused because that was what was best for his hotel-based lifestyle. He started following the diet and the cardio program religiously, and in six months he lost about 12 percent of his body fat. Suddenly, his compliance with the plan started to drop as well as his desire to assess his progress. He began to create more and more excuses, and I was shocked as he had been one of the most compliant clients I ever had up to that point. I had to analyze what had happened.

The reality of the situation was that he did not love cardio, but he had such a strong emotional connection to being overweight and wanting to change, that he would push through his dislike. When he got close to his goal, he started thinking differently about himself and lost that emotional connection that was keeping him on track. To solve this, we switched to a performance-driven goal. We started planning his workouts and slowly introducing weights. Seeing himself grow stronger and stronger, he started to see that his athleticism started to go up. He had a child that was into sports and realized that he could be a lot more involved than he ever thought. He fell in love with reaching the highest level of performance possible. The willingness and fire in his heart reignited and never wavered again. It has been years since we have trained, but he still sends me videos and pictures of the things he is accomplishing.

The answer to all goal failure is the fifth level goal. They do not have an end, meaning that if we keep working on them, they can keep improving. Examples of these goals include becoming as strong as you can, chasing certain lifts or distances in endurance, or getting your blood chemistry or sleep as optimal as you can. The point is that we feel so passionate about these goals, and we never get close enough to fall off and stop chasing them. What can be that infinite goal that you could set for yourself?

CHAPTER 5

Do It Yourself Paper Cut

Information is at our fingertips. We can, within seconds, ask Siri or Google what the cause of poor sleep is or what the components for a happy life are. With that said, as a society, we keep getting less and less sleep and getting further and further away from feelings of happiness. People still struggle with depression and anxiety even though there is all sorts of information on how to battle it. Stress is destroying lives as it is the current Black Plague of our time and one of the biggest paper cuts for our weight loss. There are two components I want to cover in this chapter. They illustrate why, although we have all the information in the world, we are not able to improve our actions.

The first component is the fact that too much of a good thing, is not a good thing, and that goes for information just the same as anything else. Searching for more information is often similar to a business owner wanting to get everything just perfect before they launch their business. They do this not realizing that they are just procrastinating. They will fail along the way, so it is essential to get going and adjust as you progress forward. Learning new information will not help you better the action plan as it just clogs up your mind with more things. This understanding is especially true now because there is so much contradicting information out there, especially when it comes to dieting. Chances are, you already know enough to get started on adopting whatever you want to change or to get on the path toward your desired destination. It is not more information that you need but the consistency of application. Once the foundation is established and you have become consistent, then it is time to search for more. I am not saying information is terrible, but that it must be consumed carefully and with a plan of application at all times.

The results of learning lead me to my second and most crucial point of why we have so much information at our fingertips yet struggle as a society in applying it. To understand this, we must dive into Bloom's Taxonomy, a concept first introduced in 1956 devised to improve communication between educators on the design of curricula and examinations. I am going to use the idea of stress management to illustrate each of the knowledge-based cognitive domains. I want to help you understand the difference between what most people know and what they must grasp in order to create change. I will run through each component utilizing weight loss as the desired outcome from learning.

Remember

It all begins with the introduction to authentic learning. This level of gathering information is the ability to remember facts and specific terminology, with no deep comprehension. It is also possessing knowledge of dealing with particular situations. For example, we learn that we need to eat fewer calories to lose weight. This fact is simple to understand and is the most foundational level of our learning experience.

Understand

After establishing the foundational knowledge, the next step is to understand the information gathered. Remembering that eating less equals losing weight does not translate into actual weight loss. Many things have to occur in between for it to happen. Comprehension involves demonstrating an understanding of facts and ideas by organizing, comparing, translating, interpreting, giving descriptions, and stating the main ideas. With weight loss, you must understand that it is not just about eating less. It is looking at an equation of how many calories you take in versus how many calories you burn during the day. This measurement determines if we are in the caloric deficit needed to burn fat. This understanding begins to separate the average consumer from someone who spent a little more time investigating the subject. Now when someone presents this information, they seem knowledgeable and worthy of our attention. However, there are four more levels left for someone to be an expert at teaching others to do something. There are vast differences between knowing something, having done it yourself, and being able to get other people to do it. This difference is where many people go wrong and follow the advice of people that only understand the material. We think they are ready to teach us, and that is a big paper cut that leads to a lot of money and time wasted.

Apply

This step requires the transference of acquired knowledge into action. Action is where most people fail. Lack of experience will lead to a lack of application, and then the desire to gain more information will come in to hide our inability to act on acquired knowledge. Often, people do not have full comprehension when they remember something and wonder why they cannot apply it. It has everything to do with how they learned the information and the depth of that learning. The difference between remembering and applying is not just in action; it has to do with being able to take information and apply it in a new way. For example, if we understand that we need to be in a caloric deficit, we know how to structure our day to increase caloric expenditure that fits our lifestyle. If you cannot commit to regular exercise, can you make it a point to park further away or take the stairs?

Could you have an alarm to move around for five minutes every hour or take walking meetings? Any of these shifts would lead to increased caloric expenditure, even if a person did not drop their intake yet. Because if they are close to where they should be, it may make all the difference. At this stage, we begin to separate novices from well-educated weight loss folks. They know that higher intensity exercise will burn more calories, so instead of just taking the stairs one step at a time, they increase movement by skipping a step as they move up. They do this to exert their body more and accomplish a more significant result with the same amount of time.

Analyze

In this step, knowledge starts to truly deepen as we make new connections between concepts. We can analyze elements in the big picture and not just at the microlevel. This newly acquired perspective would bring an understanding that not all calories are equal. They would grasp that a piece of bread worth 100 calories and a bowl of oatmeal worth 100 calories do not add up in the same way in the energy equation. The bread is probably processed and easily absorbed so the majority of those 100 calories become available and will need to be used up. Oatmeal is more complex, and energy will have to be used to break it down, so there will be less than 100 calories needed to be burned off. When you learn enough quality information and learn to analyze it to tailor it to your needs, you begin to make progress. You have reached a great place with your knowledge, but you are not finished yet.

Evaluate

The fifth component is being able to look at all the information present and decipher what information is needed and what you should ignore. Ability to solve the problem requires a depth of knowledge not yet required because there are many possible paths at this point. One must be able to, through evaluation, determine the most appropriate way to act in the situation. Often, it is not just about what is the right answer. It is more about eliminating the wrong answers so you are left with a few choices and applying the one most suitable. This process of elimination is where you earn the level of expert. From there, people can move on to the next phase: the ability to help themselves and others. This level is where great coaches separate from the rest of the pack. Trust me when I tell you that it takes years of experience to get here and why people need to put in the work to be a skilled coach. With weight loss, there are hundreds of approaches you can take, but evaluation helps you understand what is needed the most for you and your life right now. You must implement the results of your evaluation in a way that will create a winning momentum and strong habits. This stage is where all your online gurus fall away, as it is not for quick fix individuals. Being able to evaluate your health is about understanding you on the deepest level. It is about applying health correction techniques in a way that considers things like your emotions and relationships with certain foods.

Create

Now all this learning leads to the ability to create an action plan that can be executed and custom-tailored to the individual, be it for you or for a client. It is not to be confused with just making a plan because it focuses on the proper outcome versus a logical path that gets people to do something. You can create a plan at the first level of knowledge, but that plan will fall short of the desired outcome. This fact is why so many people start to fix their problems without help, but fail in the end. This failure lingers until they have put in the time to acquire all the levels needed or hired a coach to help them expedite the process.

Often, people make perfect plans on paper, and they wonder why they fail. Too much change at once will not lead you anywhere. Instead, focus on being 10 percent better each week or each month or whatever time frame you pick. It will be all you need to focus on to see success. Use this slow yet continual process and watch how you will not recognize your body, mind, and spirit after one year.

Think about how much time you have wasted over the years trying to correct your health. You may have been trying to lose weight and succeeded, but then gained it back. Perhaps you failed in the first place. How much is that time, emotional turmoil, and all the other side effects coming from failure, worth to you in money? One hundred percent of the time, if you are in this bad place, the money invested for a coach would be saved tenfold compared to what you would spend trying to do this yourself. I have never had a client that regretted spending money because they got so far, and most would pay 10 times more if they knew where they would be from the start. Why does it happen? Well, I already covered the false idea of knowledge, but it is also a fear of failure. It is not just the money but the idea that you will spend money and fail.

I am not saying that, to be successful, you must hire a coach because even great coaches will tell you that they should be working themselves out of the job by making you self-sufficient. I want to show you the steps you must go through to create the best and lasting adaptation you desire. With that said, you can only take on so much. Depending on where you are in your life right now, there are some things you may want to leave to experts. This outsourcing frees up your time to focus on what you want to become an expert in, personally.

CHAPTER 6

Relationship with Food Paper Cut

I think this might be the biggest and most common paper cut I see. Before you start to go to point B of your health journey, you must understand your point of origin. This means becoming aware of your current activities and behaviors. Most people, however, forget to analyze their relationship with food. Why is it that when you celebrate something, you usually give yourself a reward with food or drink? Why is it that when you are sad, you go toward comfort foods? The answer is one word: CONDITIONING. When you got excellent grades in school, what happened? Your parents might have taken you out for ice cream or a nice dinner. What happened when you were sad? Mom made you her famous pie that you love so much or gave you another treat. Now ask yourself: how often in your life do you feel happy and/or sad? Do you see the massive mountain you face each time you try to eat well? Do you think this is something you should blow past and just start your diet, or is it something that must be understood and broken down before you embark on the journey? I hope you see the importance of the second pathway.

We already discussed that the majority of our actions result from habitual conditioning, and we need to understand and break down those actions to replace poor responses to triggers with better ones. Sometimes it is possible to remove the trigger that caused the adverse reaction, but often it is not feasible, especially with emotional eating. Instead, you must replace the response to the trigger with one that suits your goals. To overcome this, I again encourage you to keep a food journal. I do not just mean a log of what you ate, but a record of everything that was going on around the time that you ate. If you caught yourself emotionally eating, pause and break down everything in detail in your journal by asking questions like:

- What were you doing around the time of the episode?

- Where were you at the moment when it happened and where were you before?

- What thoughts were you having then and immediately after you ate?

- What emotions were running through your mind?

- Who was with you at that time?

By doing this regularly, you will start to notice patterns. Once you identify those patterns, I recommend spending some time in deep thought around the origin of where it came from; once we understand where something came from, we can apply corrective actions to reverse or modify the behavior. The last part to add to your journal is how you feel a few hours after you had that emotional eating episode. Chances are, it is not good, and this is an important reflection to have for the next step.

From there, you need to start working on positive and negative association with food. Don't you wish you could just look at the menu and crave healthy foods rather than the bad ones? Well, that is possible through creating a more profound awareness with your nutritional choices. One of the clients I had in the past looked at eating as something negative. She associated eating food with gaining weight, so it was a very stressful and negative experience. She had an eating disorder as a kid due to being a high-level gymnast; even as an adult after years of therapy, she still had an adverse relationship with food. It took us about 15 months of continuous journaling to show her that not all the foods she ate made her feel bad. Over time, she noticed when she ate well, she felt accomplished, and when she ate poorly or not enough, her old views and feelings of judgment would come back. She realized that if she skipped a meal or made a poor choice, it was the same outcome for her emotionally. If she made good choices, all of a sudden, she felt great. What do you think that led to? Her caloric deficit went away, and meal frequency became normal, leading to stable blood sugar and the weight loss that she had been trying to achieve while starving herself for years.

If you start to understand how poor food choices impact your body, mind, and soul, you will do less and less of those actions. When you understand that good choices make you feel amazing, you naturally begin to make more of them. The goal is to shift the way you look at food. You want to get to a place where your nutrition is not about eliminating the bad, but more about chasing the good.

Remember that when we work on changing our behavior, we do not run away from a negative but run toward a positive to make long-lasting changes.

As an example, let's look at feeling sad and wanting to get ice cream. What will be the long-term effect of this? Frankly, it will lead to more sadness after the sugar rush wears off, but what if we conditioned you to go get a smoothie instead? Here is where the perfectionists of the world are going to yell that smoothies have too much sugar and are bad for weight loss, but if a person to stops eating ice cream and drinks an organic, all-natural smoothie, that is a massive win. Instead of feeling guilty, you will feel empowered because you will have appeased the sweet craving that is triggered by your brain to get more happy hormones. You put healthy nutrients into your body that gave your system the building blocks needed to feel good again. So, when having an ice cream craving, don't focus on how to avoid it as it may be stronger than your willpower. Instead, focus on getting quality nutrients quickly, ones that can give a little help with the craving but do more for you emotionally in the long run.

Emotion cannot be avoided no matter how much logic we bring into the conversation. Telling yourself that you just need to be disciplined without investigating why you feel what you feel is a huge mistake. You must truly become aware of the emotions around your food choices and figure out their origin. It is kind of like what you hear from mental health therapists. Do not push your feelings away and just push through to the finish line. You must work through and understand those feelings so you can cope with them better. It is the same thing with food even though we do not generally think that way, which is why it is such a large paper cut to our health. By working through your emotional connection with food, you will understand the trigger better and be able to replace it with a suitable response instead of the conditioned one from the past.

PART 2

Internal Health

CHAPTER 7

Result Pyramid Paper Cut

I was sitting at the fitness desk inside one of the gyms I used to work at many years ago. Two guys walked up to me and had a discussion that seemed a bit heated. They were in their late 40s and, judging by the look of their calves, they were avid cyclists. After engaging them in conversation, I was able to uncover that they were arguing over how to reduce the fat in their pectoral regions. One was saying that they needed to use testosterone, as having excess breast tissue fat for males was a sign of low testosterone. The other was saying that they needed to get more rides in during the week to burn more calories and lose weight. Which one of them do you think was right?

The answer is that neither were entirely right. In the case of these two men, after analyzing their nutrition and their weekly exercise, I knew it was the lack of recovery that was the problem. They were doing too much with their bodies, and because of that, it created a lot of stress. This stress messed with their digestion, causing a poor estrogen metabolism that kept more estrogen in their bodies than normal. Additionally, their bodies were overproducing stress response chemicals. Due to that, there were not enough building blocks to produce the right amount of sex hormones because the body uses the same resources in the production of both. This lower production caused a drop in testosterone.

Knowing the facts, what do you think I had them do to get the desired result of reducing the fat in their chests? I needed them to focus on stress reduction and had them back off on cardio and add a 20 minute cold/hot therapy in the dry sauna. They would finish a workout and go sweat for 10–20 minutes while meditating in silence. Then I had them jump in the cold pool. A month later, these guys were ecstatic from the results they saw.

What I did with them is different than what most people do. When we do not see results, we tend to do more actions that we think will get us said results. This modification is not the best course to take. When you are doing something wrong, what do you typically do? You analyze your actions and try to modify them to get the result that may be eluding you. If you are on a diet, you may do more and more things to try to lose weight, like eating fewer calories or exercising more. This change seems logical, but when it comes down to behavior change, we must remember the results pyramid. It tells us that in order to change, we do not just change the action because of the progression of results. We must start at the bottom because experience leads to a belief, a belief leads to action, and that action leads to a result.

With hundreds of my clients, I have seen them vary their actions and see no change or even less change on the scale. Why? Because they did not follow the right process of changing their beliefs by way of correcting their experience. I will use cardio for weight loss as an example here. Cardio is a great tool for weight loss, but it does not work in all situations. What if you believe that it is, in fact, the best way to lose weight because you have oversimplified the calories in/calories out equation? If you are doing it and do not see the scale change, what would you do? Well, if you are like most people, you would think you were not doing enough and keep exercising. What if the reason you are not losing weight is stress like the two gentlemen mentioned earlier? Your body does not understand the difference between running from a dinosaur and running for a workout, so doing more cardio will hurt you due to the increase in stress.

Using the results pyramid, I would change the experience for the client to get different results. Starting at the bottom of the pyramid, I would slowly take them away from cardio and add more weight training. They would begin to see a more toned body, and even though they may not have lost weight yet, their clothes might fit better. So, somebody who was a cardio junkie would begin to want more weight training. They begin to understand that it is not all about numbers on the scale, as body fat is ultimately what makes us healthy and unhealthy. We can get better without actually losing weight on the scale. This improvement creates consistency with weight training, and before you know it the pounds start to melt off as the initial increase in muscle mass slows down and the fat burn catches up.

There are many examples, but the biggest point is to expand your perspective on your options by trying new experiences. The same thing can apply to say, recovery workouts. Often, I have seen people get diminishing results from exercise. They try so hard that they do not give their body enough time to recover. I tell my clients that it is like trying to learn a second language by constantly consuming new information and not giving your mind time to process it. This way will not work. So, I can't just advise people to back off, as their beliefs from their experience tell them they must go harder to accomplish results. Instead, I must slowly change their experience. Maybe it is not by first getting them to back off and reduce what they do, but by adding additional recovery sessions. By utilizing things like floatation therapy and dry sauna recovery, they start to notice belly fat reduction due to lowered stress. Experience leads them to a more open mind, and it begins to change their belief system, leading to more recovery actions. As the results continue, they naturally begin to shift to a more balanced workout regimen. They realize that planning their recovery is just as important as planning hardcore workouts for their health and weight loss.

Do not commit the paper cut of doing more of the same thing and expecting a different result. At the same time, do not simply vary your actions without understanding the origins of them. Instead, create an experience that leads to the right belief and changes your actions to ones that accomplish results. This is how long-lasting habits are created and what I focus so much on in my #10PercentFITTER Method.

CHAPTER 8

Water Paper Cut

We are mainly made up of water, yet so many people fail to drink enough of it. We all know someone who is obsessive about keeping every fluid in their car in check and topped off. However, we do not usually see this kind of focus on maintaining the fluids of our body. Lack of water intake is a massive paper cut that causes things like reduced energy, making poor dietary options, and increased stress in the body. Think about how long your engine will run if it lacks oil or how well your car will work without the coolant liquid being at full level. The same thing occurs in your human engine.

Water plays many vital functions that you do not usually consider when it comes to remembering how much you need to be drinking. It plays importance with seven vital roles in our body: it transports, dissolves, cleans, reacts, pads, and regulates temperature.

The transporting function of water is its ability to move things to and from the cells of our body. It transports things like nutrients and oxygen, which are extremely important for our body to grow and repair itself. Water also carries messages from our hormones to the rest of our system. It also helps remove waste out of the body, like carbon dioxide. The dissolving function is for breaking down things like sugar and certain minerals. Water flushes vital filtering organs like the kidneys and liver, which remove toxins from our bodies.

Additionally, water plays an important role in the chemical reactions in our body. It also helps with lubrication in your joints, digestive tract, and lungs so your body feels and functions better for you. Water also provides padding within the joints and helps you regulate your body temperature. Can you imagine what it would be like in the heat if you could not sweat? And these are just some of the reasons why you need to ensure you have adequate daily water intake.

I cover functions of water because you need to understand why it is important, which should help you create a habit around it. The amount which I recommend is half of your body weight, in pounds, consumed as water, in ounces, per day. I have tried many methods to ensure I hit this number, and I have uncovered that the biggest paper cut is having a small container, like a typical sized water bottle. The problem lies in us forgetting to refill the bottle and falling too far behind our intake for the day. What I have found personally and with my clients is that when we have a large container, it makes it clear the amount of water we have drunk in a day. We do much better with holding ourselves accountable by having this visual reminder. I prefer glass bottles as they are clear and plastic-free. I drink my first half by lunch and work on getting the second half done by dinner, so I am not drinking too much liquid before bed.

The other reason why water is essential is the research coming out on the increase in weight loss during the time that people are dieting.

In this study[1], researchers told a mix of different people to come into the lab twice. The first time they were to eat as much food as they wanted. The second time they were to drink 500 mL of water

1. Dennis EA, Dengo AL, Comber DL, Flack KD, Savla J, Davy KP, Davy BM. Water consumption increases weight loss during a hypocaloric diet intervention in middle-aged and older adults. Obesity (Silver Spring). 2010 Feb;18(2):300-7.

and then eat as much as they wanted. The researchers wanted to see whether people would eat less if they drank water before a meal. After the initial lab visit, all participants went on a diet that permitted 1,200 kcal per day for women and 1,500 kcal per day for men. Note, I do not personally recommend these caloric intakes.

Everybody was on the same diet, but half the participants had a secret pre-meal supplement: 500 mL of water.

Before each of their three meals, the water group drank 500 mL of water, and then they could eat. Twelve weeks later, at the end of the study, all the participants did the water drinking test again. Over the three months, the water group dropped 4.4 percent of body fat (from 39.9 percent to 36.5 percent) and 5.4 kg of total fat, while the non-water group only dropped 1.1 percent of body fat (from 41.0 percent to 38.9 percent) and 3.3 kg of total fat. So, the bottom line here is that drinking two cups of water before a meal will keep you hydrated, fuller, and may even boost your metabolism.

Another big paper cut is drinking unfiltered water from the tap or stored in plastic water bottles for an extended time. This toxic exposure builds up chemicals in your body not meant for your system and creates all sorts of havoc, from behavior issues to hormonal imbalances. I already mentioned that I use a glass bottle and elimination of toxins is just one of the reasons, helping the environment is another big one as well. One of the things I do when helping people overcome estrogen dominance is the elimination of the use of plastic. Using a lot of plastic before you get to your mid-40s will lead to a tough road of recovery.

In summary, before you begin to diet and make massive changes, make sure you are hitting that minimal water intake.

CHAPTER 9

Resting Metabolism Paper Cut

Metabolism is so incredibly complex and yet you always hear it grossly simplified to two states: fast or slow. Your thyroid has much to do with it, but many other factors affect metabolism as well. One of the most significant health paper cuts that leads to unmaintained results is not paying attention to your metabolism at rest.

In the U.S., the average male will burn about 1,800 calories in a single day at rest while the average female will burn about 1,400. Those numbers are resting metabolic rates, often abbreviated as RMR. This means that if we laid in bed and did absolutely nothing, we would burn that many calories. In a tough one-hour workout, you can burn anywhere from 500–1,000 calories, yet your body does almost double that at rest. Understanding your metabolism at rest is an important aspect of health and essential for weight loss maintenance once you have achieved the goal. I have helped people raise their metabolism by 300–750 calories daily by focusing on burning more of the right fuel in larger quantities. What is always the right fuel? Fat. Why? Because we have so much of it available to us in our body's storage.

Let's play this out to illustrate the point. Say you were burning 1,400 calories at rest and over the course of a year we changed that to 2,000 calories. Those 600 calories could be all the difference. Say before you were slowly gaining weight, and now, due to this increase, instead of being over by 100 calories every day, your intake is under 500 calories. For simple math, we will say that 3,500 calories equal one pound of fat. So, over the course of a week without doing anything extra, you could be losing a pound. This adaptation is the true solution of how to lose weight and keep it off, as well as having more energy overall.

The other change with resting metabolism can come from adjusting what our body uses for fuel. At any given point, you are burning fat and sugar, which provides the energy the body needs. A healthy adult should be using up about 80 percent fat and 20 percent sugar at rest. Due to the many paper cuts covered in this book, this ratio can change drastically. Imagine that now you are burning 60 percent fat and 40 percent carbohydrate. Well, over the course of a day for an average female, that can be a difference of 280 calories of fat not being consumed and for a male it can be around 360 calories. So that means in anywhere between a week and two weeks, you could be gaining or maintaining pounds of fat just by these ratios varying. This formula is why not all calories are equal, as they create this kind of change to our metabolism.

So what do we do to impact our resting metabolism to get the desired results and keep them for years to come? There are many things you can do, but I will cover the three major techniques that will help you to optimize your fuel usage.

Eat more fat and fewer carbohydrates, especially the refined ones.

Your body is the most advanced piece of machinery in the world. It is built for survival and adjusts its function based on the inputs provided. I once spoke with a nutritionist for the U.S. National Triathlon

Team, and I wanted to pick his brain on metabolism. He told me that he could help endurance athletes change their performance faster through modifying their diet than modifying their workouts. Why? Because if your body gets more of a particular fuel source consistently throughout the day, it learns to adjust by burning that fuel more. He was focused on improving an athlete's active metabolism, but the same phenomenon affects the resting metabolism too. This adaptation is why the Keto diet is so popular. People consume a much higher percentage of fat than sugar at rest, and it leads to increased percentages of fat utilization that can cause weight loss or make weight loss easier to maintain. Now remember I am not an advocate of diets, so I am merely showing you why the Keto diet works.

Increase your VO2

Your VO2 is the measurement of how much your body can consume oxygen. Cardio, for example, is not just good for burning calories. If you do it in proper intensities, you can increase how much oxygen your body pulls in at rest. The more oxygen you have available, the easier it is for your body to consume fat. Often, there is not enough oxygen, so your percentage of fat fuel to sugar fuel skews in the wrong direction. A big paper cut that people make here is either not doing enough cardio or doing too much cardio for too long a time, but I will cover this more in later chapters. This amazing property of our body is why I have my clients do breathing exercises in their off times. Breathwork enhances the way they breathe and, in turn, improves their oxygen intake and utilization. This modification leads to weight loss and gives them a better stress response throughout the day.

Increase lean muscle mass

Usually when I bring this modification up, especially to women, I get pushback. Why? Because people see fitness magazines and assume increased muscle mass means bulk. I make a joke in this case and ask the person if they drive a car. When they say yes, I ask them if they are afraid of becoming a racecar driver. It's the same principle with lifting weights. Just because you lift weights a few times a week does not mean you are going to look like one of the people in those magazines. Chances are, you will only add a bit of muscle mass because bulking up is a prolonged process that requires a lot of consistency and extra calories. A man, under excellent conditions, can build muscle somewhere around 1 to 2 lbs. per month and for a woman, somewhere between 0.5 to 1 lbs. per month. This rate slows down with more exercise, as the body adjusts to the applied stimulus over time, so the extra 5 to 10 pounds of muscle you add will not bulk you. This extra muscle will actually tighten you because it is much denser than fat. The other benefit is that for every pound of muscle that you add, your body will burn more calories at rest in order to maintain that muscle. This increase positively impacts your resting metabolism, not by 50 calories per pound but more like 6–35 calories.

The important part is that you are moving toward a more functional metabolism and not running away from food. This shift in thinking is how you break the diet cycle and optimize your body.

CHAPTER 10

Treating Symptoms Paper Cut

About eight years ago, I found a new client who was willing to invest and do whatever it took to lose the weight she had gained over the last couple of decades. Three months later and $6,000 out of her pocket, she had only lost 6 pounds when she wanted to lose 70. You can imagine her frustration with having to pay $1,000 per pound lost. She would log all her food, do the appropriate intensity of cardio, and was measured by a computer. She received nutrition coaching and worked out for three days with me and three days on her own. Yet we only saw a tiny result. She was blaming me for being a bad trainer, and I was blaming her because I thought she had to be lying with her food log, as it made no sense.

We battled back and forth for about a month until, finally, I learned about blood chemistry and how it can be a roadblock. She had a comprehensive blood panel performed, and it uncovered why the weight was not coming off. Her body was having issues with burning fat from having too much negative estrogen and digestive issues that were creating inflammation. Additionally, she had sleep problems due to high stress that I was not aware of because she thought it was normal. So, immediately we shifted focus away from weight loss and toward correcting those deep-rooted issues. Before you know it, the weight started melting off at a rate of 10 lbs. per month. Why did this happen?

Weight gain or the inability to lose weight is a symptom from our body. It is not the problem in and of itself, even though it may be the most significant symptom you want to correct. Trying to fix symptoms without correcting the root issues is like rolling two balls up a hill simultaneously. You push one for a bit and get ahead, but the minute you let it go to focus on the other, you end up in the same place you started. We must stop these paper cuts of only attempting to solve symptoms. By addressing the root cause, you learn to go with the flow to create permanent change that gets results tomorrow, which maintains them a year from now and does not negatively impact your health 10 years down the road.

When you focus on the symptoms, you do not do your due diligence concerning your starting point. You run full speed ahead without evaluating if there are better practices for your body. Yes, they may help, but how much and at what cost? Everything has what is called an opportunity cost. It means that by investing time into one thing, you are taking away time from other things you could be doing. When you use methods that are marginally intended for your actual problem, you end up wasting a lot of time. Your improvement is only a fraction of what you could see if you had taken actions that were meant specifically for you instead. What if, during this time, you lost motivation? What if your environment changed and it was harder to focus on yourself? When you are on a personal health journey, you need to ensure that, when the time is right, you act on it in the most precise way or the opportunity could pass you by.

So how do you find out your starting point? One word: ASSESSMENT. Depending on the symptoms, there are plenty of tests out there that will give you an idea of where to start. I carry a bunch that I use with my clients on my website, but there are even more. For example, if you are not sleeping well and think that stress may be the culprit, I would order an at-home saliva collection kit. This kit will let you know how your stress response is doing, and from that, you can create a plan of what behaviors you need to change as well as what supplements would be best.

If you feel that your digestion is poor, a great place to start is to see a gastroenterologist as there are a battery of tests they can run. However, they do not always give you an answer. Your problems could be due to sensitivities that I will cover later, and you may need to do an elimination diet. If that is too hard right now, then order a food sensitivity panel, which is not the same as a food allergy test. These tests are not covered by insurance, but it often uncovers what may be missed by the doctors, unless they happen to be naturopaths.

For metabolism, you can do what is called a metabolic assessment. There are two versions of it. One tells you your active metabolism and things like at what intensity you burn fat best and at what intensity you stop burning fat. It can also tell you how the calories, fat, and sugar are being used at each intensity. This will uncover all the opportunities you have to fix your metabolism through cardio. If you want to figure out your resting metabolism, there is a resting version of this test. With both, you get hooked up to an oxygen mask, and a machine calculates how your body is doing.

There are lots of ways to uncover where your starting point is, but it is incredibly essential that you investigate your symptoms before jumping into a program. Time is a precious resource, and I do not want you to waste it. You must understand the root of the problem and start there instead of treating each symptom like a leaf on a tree.

CHAPTER 11

Sleep Paper Cut

I wish I could get a dollar for every time I heard, "I'm fine, I function great on five to six hours of sleep a day." These kinds of statements have become common because of the "success" mindset that is perpetuated by popular culture. Many people say that if you want something, you need to work 12–16 hours a day to make it happen. When you add in other life commitments, you don't have enough time for health and cut out time from your sleep. The thing that I want to remind people is that you can make all the money in the world, but if you are like my dad and die at a very early age, you won't even be able to enjoy it.

I met one of my clients because I was working with his wife. He traveled 75 percent of the time and was a high-level executive for a large corporation. He slept maybe five hours a night on average. He had a significant amount of belly fat even though he was working out regularly and had very little fat in other areas. His diet was better than average because he was well educated health-wise The minute I saw him, I knew that stress was the culprit. We always carry body fat disproportionately when we have certain hormonal imbalances and stress tends to centralize it. With that said, it was a challenge to convince him that his sleep was one of the reasons for his stressed state. Why? Because he had high energy in the morning and only got tired midday, and he blamed that on general fatigue because it had been that way for many years.

I have mentioned that common does not equal normal, and that goes for society overall and the individual. Just because it was common for him to experience life that way does not mean it was normal as far as his health goes. We need contrast to compare things, and when the change takes over a decade to set in, we forget what our best feels like. He did not see how his memory and his ability to focus had been hindered because of stress and lack of sleep. And he did not connect his belly fat to that one bad habit.

So, what did we do to correct it? Before I could even begin to help him fix his sleep problem, we had to create awareness. I could have told him all of the things he was doing wrong and given him the solutions, but if he did not believe that he had a problem, he would not have been compliant long term. Think of your health journey as if you are driving down a road. Each time you go through an intersection, you need a green light, or an understanding of the full implications of what you are dealing with. If you go through on a yellow light, you at least grasp the general concept and believe in it. However, if you blow through a red light without having a foundational understanding, it can derail your entire journey from that point forward. This is one of the many components in creating long-lasting habits with your health.

To start, I had my client set an alarm that would remind him that he had an hour to finish up his evening and get ready for bed. The focus was on just that action without any expectations. We set a behavior goal and worked on it for 30 days, overcoming setbacks. From there, each month we worked on adding sleep hygiene techniques one at a time in order to build up his evening routine. One of the reasons he was staying up late was that his body was not winding down until after midnight due to stress. By improving his sleep hygiene and managing his stress, within three months we were able to get him falling asleep within five minutes before 10 p.m. The components of his sleep hygiene were as follows.

We limited stimulants, like coffee, to where he could only have them up until 12 p.m. Stimulants impact our circadian rhythm and often are one of the reasons why people have a hard time winding down.

We limited his nightcaps. He used to drink a couple of beers at night to relax, but after I showed him how it was hurting his sleep, he started to cut back and eventually only drank socially. Alcohol severely impacts vital REM sleep and increases the levels of a stress hormone called cortisol. If you struggle with quitting this habit, start by switching to red wine, as it has some positive benefits, and then eventually let the alcohol go as you no longer need it to wind down.

We had him increase his vegetable intake at dinner. By eating more veggies, your body will increase serotonin and melatonin production. These two neurotransmitters are responsible for calming our body down and getting us ready for sleep. I worked on getting rid of some of the simple carbs he was eating and adding veggies that he found fun ways to cook. Variety is essential, as you do not want to get bored with what you are eating.

We worked on decreasing his blue light exposure before bed. He would always work on his computer at night, but the adjustment was necessary as blue light negatively impacts sleep. Light is a significant regulator of our natural sleep, and if we get a lot of it at night, it makes our body think it is not time for bed. This is also why it is great to get some sunlight first thing in the morning. I had him install a red light filter on his phone and computer that blocked out all the blue light, which still gave him the ability to do some work without too much of a negative effect on his sleep cycle. I also had him turn down the lights in the house for the last two hours of his day.

We lowered the bedroom temperature. He lived in Arizona, so this was an easy change for him. I asked him to sleep at a temperature of 68 degrees instead of the 70 he was used to, and he felt cozier while he slept.

Last, but most certainly not least, we optimized his sleeping environment by covering up all the little lights in the room. Believe it or not, some people are so light-sensitive that the standby light on televisions can negatively impact sleep. He covered up his TV light, the smoke alarm light, and made sure that no external lights were seeping into the room by switching to blackout curtains.

It was incredible what these changes did for him so he became convinced of the positive impact sleep could have on his overall health. It was not about telling him but having him experience it. Remember the results pyramid. If we want to change the outcome, we don't just push new actions. We must change our beliefs through experience first.

Those beliefs will lead to new actions, eliciting different results. For example, that same client eventually started meditating and doing yoga after noticing these changes.

If sleep is a problem for you, modifying your lifestyle is one way to help. Some people, however, have no issue falling asleep but can be awakened by the drop of a pin. This often comes from an unexpected source: your blood sugar regulation. If your body has poor blood sugar regulation, you end up having big crashes at night that come with a chemical spike that signals your body to get more energy. You wake up feeling like you have to go to the bathroom because you have a bit of urine in your bladder, but you do not realize it was a chemical response that woke you.

To see if this might be the case, run this little experiment. Eat 1/2 cup of browned sweet potatoes right before you go to bed and see if your sleep improves. The carbohydrates will do two big things for you. Because of the complexity of the sweet potato, your body will take time to break it down, and it will give your body higher levels of blood sugar than you would have otherwise. If you notice better sleep, then you know that you must work on your blood sugar regulation.

Perhaps you fall asleep easily and wake up super early, and you can't go back to sleep because you have so much energy. This may be a great thing if you like to get into the gym at 3 a.m. and start your day with exercise, but only if you can get seven to eight hours of sleep per night. Why? Because of the reasons behind your excess energy. Your body could be under stress, and your cortisol levels could be higher than normal in the morning. Because cortisol is a fight-or-flight hormone, it gives you energy for increased performance. However, there are many long-term problems if this is a chronic occurrence. Your body won't be able to handle excess energy in the morning forever, and 10–20 years down the road, or even sooner, you will have a crash. That crash can take up to 1.5 years of medication and therapy to get out of, so it is not worth the risk.

If that is the case and your body is overly stressed, my best advice for you is mindfulness. Now if you do not believe in Eastern medicine, I am not telling you to meditate. I personally believe meditation is the best medicine, but that should not disqualify you from being mindful. If you want to try some guided meditation, I have some recordings on my YouTube channel and website that will help you achieve better sleep. If you remain uncomfortable with meditation, I still want you to understand mindfulness. It is a time where you are not anywhere but the exact moment you are in. Try going for a walk in a park and instead of worrying about what is to come or what has passed, observe the wind whistling through the leaves and smell the fragrance of the freshly trimmed grass. Feel every step as it happens and notice all the processes happening in your body that automatically create that movement. Maybe you are religious and could spend moments of solitude praying. The same thing should be accomplished in prayer as in meditation: the complete devotion to the moment. Reading can be useful, but if light interferes, it can be problematic at night. If that is the case, read in the afternoons for a similar positive effect.

Remember that if sleep is a problem, you can do an assessment to test your stress and sleep. The point is that you have the tools to overcome sleep issues. Some of these techniques you can implement yourself, and for others, you may need help from people like me. Even if you get six hours of sleep each night instead of seven to eight, it is as if you did not sleep a whole day during a week. That strain on your health is one of the biggest reasons why not sleeping well is such a sizable paper cut. It all compounds and shows up down the road in ways we cannot anticipate.

CHAPTER 12

Distracted Life Paper Cut

Yesterday is history, tomorrow is a mystery, and today is a gift; that is why we call it the present. When we consider this statement, we begin to see how important being present is. We are not promised tomorrow, so the million thoughts that continually come into your head are not going to serve you. Is there time to plan? Yes, there is a dedicated time to decide what you will do in the future. With that said, sitting there pondering all day long what has not occurred is not useful for everyone. On the other hand, yesterday is gone, and we cannot do anything about it. Should we reflect and learn a lesson? Absolutely, but that does not mean we should be contemplating what happened all the time and letting that preoccupy our minds and distract us from what is going on right then.

What are some of the paper cuts that come from not being present? First, your mind is continuously taxed, and it puts a lot of stress on your system, even though you may not be thinking about anything particularly stressful. You must remember that your body can react the same way to a thought as it can to something happening in real life. When you are under constant stress, your body struggles to regulate its response; instead of being able to respond appropriately on a scale of 1-10, every stressful thought and action creates a 10 out of

10 response. By not being present, you can push your body to being on constant red alert.

From there, we need to identify that not being present impacts social skills as well. Instead of paying attention to what is being said, you are focusing on your response or thinking about something from the past that may connect to the conversation. What will that do? It will cause you to have poor body language that conveys to the other person that what they are saying is not essential. We know that having a good support system is important, so do not burn those bridges because you are a poor communicator not operating in the present.

Do you get bored of eating the same thing and doing the same kinds of workouts? If you are like most people, the answer is yes. What does this have to do with being present? To have variety, we need to be creative, and when we are not present, that creativity diminishes. When we are high with a stress response, we are sharper and more analytical. But when our stress response hormones are low, we are more creative. We already established that being preoccupied with the past or the future leads to higher levels of stress in our body. Now we can tie that into our ability to not have tunnel vision and being creative with our nutrition and workouts.

When you are present, you are much more playful. This translates into overall enjoyment of the activities you are doing. Let's be honest, when you are just starting your health journey, exercising and learning to eat well *and* managing your internal health is not that fun. You need all the help you can get, and if there is a way for your body to feel more excited about these activities, you will be more amenable over the long term and see more success.

Ultimately, you must remember that when your stress hormones are up, your ability to burn fat goes down. This knowledge is the most crucial reason for needing to be present in your life.

There are many tricks to improving your focus, like meditation and other stress management techniques, but for now, I want to cover three that do not require much time. The first one is the way that you breathe. How often do you stop and pay attention to how you are breathing? I want you to pause right now. You have been reading for a bit, so your breath may be nice and smooth. In other moments of your life, pause and observe. Chances are you will notice that the breath is often shallow and choppy and is more in the top of your chest rather than your belly. By regularly monitoring your breath and slowing it down to use more of the diaphragm, you will notice your body calm down and become more aware of sensations in you and your environment. I know that overweight people can be self-conscious about their midsection and often like to pull it in, keeping more air up in the chest. We are not meant to breathe this way, and beyond the stress, this action also causes movement problems and, eventually, pain. You may think you look better by sucking in your gut, but is it worth the negative side effects?

The next way to practice being present is by eating slowly. Try this exercise the next time you have a meal. Observe what your thoughts are and journal how you feel during and after that meal. During the next meal, slow down and do not allow your mind to wander by implementing two techniques. Try to chew 15 times each time you take a bite, and afterwards, set down your utensils and look around a bit. Focus on the sensation of the food. Notice the flavor, the texture, and your presence in the space around you. Then journal about it and compare the two states. This subjective information will give you proof as to why it is a good idea to be present while eating.

Finally, observe the details around you, don't just see something and categorize it as a random object. Instead of just seeing a tree, notice how the leaves move in the wind and all the other finer details that make up a tree. Instead of just listening to a person, notice their respiration rate, their facial expressions, and all the tiny fluctuations of their voice.

None of these techniques are going to require you to invest more time, but when done with consistency and with practice, they become fantastic resources in helping you stay more present. You can avoid the paper cuts mentioned above and, most importantly, always maximize your ability to burn fat as fuel.

The biggest reason we are challenged by remaining present is that we do not categorize our thoughts properly. How much time do you think you spend worrying about things you cannot control? If you start to journal these thoughts, you will be amazed at what a tremendous amount of time it is. When we fixate on a thought, it is as if our body is experiencing it. We become stressed from merely thinking.

Writing down your worries is a best practice I call "The Three Stress Buckets." As you sit there with your journal, write down the thoughts that have been preoccupying your mind. Perhaps they are of things that have happened or things that are coming up tomorrow or later in the week. Next, put them in one of the three categories.

Bucket one is where you place things that you directly control. Those things are not dependent on anyone else but you. They are dependent on you taking action. Two examples are what time you set your alarm for in the morning and what time you lay down to go to bed at night.

Bucket two is where you place all the things that you can influence. Those things are dependent on you taking a specific action, but also involve another component. It could be someone else making a decision or an outcome based on forces outside yourself. An example would be how you get your kids to behave at the grocery store. You decide whether or not you give them sugar or if you give in to their requests for toys. Ultimately, you know that you cannot control if they end up having a meltdown or not. When you become aware of these thoughts, I want you to write down what you directly controlled in the situation. Whether it happened before or is yet to come, write out all the actions you can control and let go of all of the rest.

Finally, bucket three is where you place things that you cannot control or influence at all. They are completely independent of you, and you cannot impact them one way or another. The simplest example of that is traffic or the weather. How often do you stress about things like that? By reflecting on and identifying all three of these types of thoughts, you allow for better awareness in the moment they happen. In turn, you overcome the unhelpful thoughts quicker and return to being present.

CHAPTER 13

Recovery Paper Cut

She was an owner of a large real estate agency. She had been fit her entire life and was even the owner of a gym with multiple locations back in the '90s. She taught health classes and nutrition education. She came to me because, just like many of you, she had stopped seeing results in her later years. She would work harder and harder, with more commitment than most of us show, and only ended up gaining weight in the process.

I could hear it in her voice and see it in her body language from the moment we sat down: frustration. This meeting was only five years ago, and I had not been actively working with clients for a few years because I was more in the space of teaching other health coaches how to get results for people. During this meeting, for some reason, something clicked in my head that made a big life change for me. I decided I wanted to help her and get back into health coaching, just not work with everyone. I wanted to focus on people like her, those that did the work but struggled to get consistent and sustainable results from the custom practices one finds in health coaching.

Her diet was clean, her workouts would often happen twice a day, and she was very active with her high-level soccer playing sons. But month after month, the scale did not move. By looking at her, I noticed that she carried a disproportionate amount of fat in her midsection compared to the rest of her body. The problem that she had is the paper cut I want to discuss in this chapter, and it is one that many are committing.

In the sports and fitness industry, you will hear the word overtraining a lot. It means that a person will get fewer results by doing more because their body is physically overstressed. It is tough to prove this concept to people because mentally, they could feel fine and think that stress is not a significant roadblock for them. However, without them realizing, it is silently wreaking havoc on their system. Yes, my client was overdoing her workouts, but what we do not consider is the workload and the amount of stress we impose on our bodies in our everyday lives. Your job, your relationships, your family, and your busy daily schedule all stress your body out even if you do not find those things especially stressful.

The reality of the situation is that there is no overtraining but rather under recovering. The same thing goes for health and fitness as it does for everyday life. You can work and go as hard as you want under one condition. You must give your body enough time to recover from the activity. If you put in an hour at the gym doing some light work, you could probably return for a second workout if you slept well the night before. However, if you just did a grueling hour where you can barely crawl away from the fitness floor, you may need a full day or potentially two days before doing another hard workout like that.

The concept of overtraining is not common knowledge yet, but it is starting to become more widely known. Say you just worked a long day at the office, and then ran home to take one kid to soccer practice and the second kid to gymnastics. In between all that, you had to run and get groceries for dinner. Then you had to knock out lunch prep for the kids for the next day. Your partner is at work

10–12 hours a day, and as much as they want to, they are not able to help out. Then you get a late-night phone call about an emergency that you have to handle first thing in the morning. It takes forever to fall asleep knowing what you have to face, and then the next day, you must rinse and repeat. Doing this for consecutive days without giving your body rest is the same as doing grueling workouts multiple times a day without taking breaks. The body is going to eventually wear out from the stress and start gaining fat by only wanting to burn sugar.

This situation was the case for my client. To help her, I had to teach her how to recover better. Notice I did not say back off. She was not willing to slow down, so I had her meditating, doing flotation therapy, and the hot sauna/cold plunge routine post workouts. I also had her eat regular meals to get her blood sugar stable as that is another stressor on the body. She did not cook, so we had her set up a meal delivery service.

When a month went by without results, the client was angry and ready to stop. I, knowing the process well, asked her to give me one more month, and if it did not work, I would cover the next month's costs myself. This challenge gave her enough reassurance to keep going. Guess what happened? First, she told me how she was feeling much better and more focused. And as she came in for her regular two week checkups, she noticed the weight was coming off, and the inches were falling off as well. Although she was doing significantly fewer workouts, as we redistributed some of that time to recovery activities, she saw results for the first time in years. Just a few short months down the road, she ended up in better shape than she had been in over 15 years. I was so proud of all of her hard work but prouder of her learning to let go a bit and discover the benefits of recovery.

One of the biggest breakthroughs came when she began to understand that stress was not just in her mind. Being a very resilient person, she would brush things off. Our minds, however, are much stronger than our bodies. This is a big paper cut that many of you make because you think that stress cannot be a root cause as you don't actually feel very stressed. Remember, many types of stressors can plague the body but may not be perceived as much by the mind.

From watching this client succeed, I fell in love with the idea of helping high achievers stay at their peak level of performance while maintaining their energy, physique, and life fulfillment. I saw how she was able to continue being amazing in all areas of her life, all while taking on a healing health journey. With proper pacing and supercharged recovery methods, you can do that too. Had my client not controlled the specific areas of her life that she did, she would not have been as successful. The greatest area of control was her recovery and the amount of time she invested in it.

There are two methods of recovery that I recommend in expediting the process. These methods are to recovery as steroids are to the body when you are trying to build muscle. The first method, and probably my favorite, is float spas. You enter a small pod, and the space is filled with about two feet of water in which you lay down and relax. Because the water has upwards of 1,000 lbs. of dissolved Epsom salt, it is very buoyant. Your body becomes suspended in the water, without touching anything. The complete deprivation of your senses combined with large quantities of magnesium absorption make this an ultra-therapeutic experience. You come close to sleeping, and the experience does wonders for your brain in recovering from burnout.

My second go-to recovery method is temperature therapy, which I do in many ways. Being born in Russia, my father introduced me to this as a very young boy. It was said that this practice was good for improving immunity. It is true because, by being more present and improving stress response, you do precisely that. We used to sit in superhot steam rooms and lightly whip each other with leaves and tree branches. Then, once we could not take the heat, we would either run out and jump into a pile of snow or the cold water of a lake or the sea.

Now, I do this method with a dry sauna or steam room. I prefer the dry sauna to the steam room as it is has the ability to get much hotter. I stay in the dry sauna until I become uncomfortable, about 10–20 minutes, and then I jump into a cold pool or shower. It is very rejuvenating and great for detoxing as well. Cryotherapy chambers are some of my favorite places to recover as well. If those are not available or if I do not want to spend the money, two 20 lb. bags of ice in a bathtub can do the trick. I jump in for about 10 minutes, but I do not submerge my feet and hands until the end. Trust me when I say that you are never more present than when you are in a tub of ice; nothing else but survival through that moment matters.

I hope you see all the great ways that, even if you do not have a lot of time, you can keep your body recovered. Because there is always a way. Set the constraints and find the inputs that work for your lifestyle and goals.

CHAPTER 14

Paper Cut of the Gut Membrane

One of my clients walked into her first appointment wearing clothing that was tight in all the places except the midsection. As I put her on the body fat scale, I saw that she carried all of her fat there. Naturally, I thought stress was the problem as the midsection is where stress hormones like to pack on the pounds. After investigating her life during the intake process, I realized she did not have much stress. I was confused because all the symptoms said that stress was the issue. When I started digging more, I realized her body was inflamed, and she reported being very bloated. Then it hit me: her stress was not mental. Her stress was coming from her gut. After taking her through a digestive questionnaire, I realized that she had all the symptoms of a leaky gut.

This meeting was ten years ago, and at that time, the term "leaky gut" was not widely accepted and understood. She looked at me in confusion and said, "So you are saying my gut sprung a leak and is leaking inside my body?" Understanding her bewilderment, I explained that it was happening on a cellular level and not on the scale she may be imagining in her mind. Our stomach has a lining that acts as a defense system, and its job is to keep bad bacteria and food that is not fully digested out of the bloodstream. There are small junctures that, when functioning correctly, pass the right things through and keep the wrong things out. People damage that lining in many ways, like with poor nutrition, too much stress, or toxic exposure. At that point, it is no longer doing its job effectively. An increase in intestinal permeability causes all sorts of ill effects, the main one being inflammation. Leaky gut, in combination with poor food absorption, can halt weight loss no matter what other external factors are present and the reason why it is such a big paper cut.

The list of possible conditions stemming from the leaky gut is vast, but here are some that researchers have identified:

- ALS (Lou Gehrig's disease)
- Alzheimer's disease
- Anxiety and depression
- Attention deficit hyperactivity disorder (ADHD)
- Autism
- Celiac disease and non-celiac gluten sensitivity
- Chronic fatigue syndrome
- Crohn's disease
- Fibromyalgia
- Hashimoto's disease
- Irritable bowel syndrome (IBS)
- Lupus
- Metabolic syndrome
- Migraines
- Multiple sclerosis

- Non-alcoholic fatty liver disease

- Parkinson's disease

- Polycystic ovary syndrome

- Restless legs syndrome

- Rheumatoid arthritis

- Yeast overgrowth

Leaky gut has clear symptoms so look through these and see if any fit your experience. Then you can investigate if leaky gut may be a roadblock for your results. Some symptoms include:

- You have an autoimmune disease

- You have Crohn's disease or ulcerative colitis

- You suffer from IBS

- You get seasonal allergies

- You have soft bowel movements on a regular basis

- You do not have a daily bowel movement

- You get sick often, three to four times per year

- You know you have struggled with yeast, *Candida*, or fungal issues

- You crave sweets and/or bread

- You struggle with skin conditions

- You have a high level of stress in your life

- You get gas and/or feel bloated

- You get heartburn and indigestion

- You have thyroid issues and a slow metabolism

- You have a history of antibiotics or other prescription medications

If you answered "yes" to four or more of these, chances are, you may be facing a leaky gut. This will make it incredibly hard, if not impossible, to lose weight. You could be eating properly and exercising regularly and still not see the scale move or feel your energy levels and sense of well-being improving. So, what must you do? Remember, this book is not a comprehensive outline on how to fix every issue, so I will not go into great detail. However, I want you to be aware enough to ask better questions about the habits that apply to you. With that said, there are five main leaky gut types, and you could have a combination of them.

Candida gut is one of the most common types you will see, affecting more than 70 percent of Americans. It is related to yeast overgrowth and often comes from having too much yeast and refined sugar in your diet. Many severely overweight people have this as a problem.

Then we have the Gastric gut, which is caused by a small intestinal overgrowth of bacteria. Also known as SIBO, it is a medical condition in which a person has more bacteria in their small intestine than normal. SIBO is a complication of other digestive conditions: IBS, Crohn's disease, and celiac disease.

Then we have the Immune gut. This one ties into food allergies, intolerances, and sensitivities. It is important to understand that allergies and sensitivities are very different. Your doctor could be telling you that you have no known allergies. Yet your gut could be having all sorts of problems. Why does this happen? Because sensitivities, the lowest level of impact on the body from food, are not easily identifiable. This is due to the response taking a long time to occur. The body can have a mild reaction up to 72 hours after the food was ingested, so it is challenging to connect the problem with the source.

The Toxic gut is another form of leaky gut. It comes from being exposed to too much toxicity, which is why I am not a fan of alcohol. It is not just about the sugars and the calories. The bigger problem is the toxicity our body has to work through when we drink. This type of gut problem can lead to gallbladder diseases, skin conditions, and chronic liver disease.

Last but not least, the Stressed gut. This one is terrifying to me because it is difficult to catch. Chronic stress wreaks havoc on your system, and your digestive tract is not immune. When you are always stressed, digestion is not one of the places your body wants to give resources to, as it is prioritizing survival. This will cause negative effects on your adrenal glands, kidneys, thyroid, and sex hormones, as well as lead to fatigue.

You can see a specialist where they will run tests to see which of these situations you are facing and design a good plan to reverse the problem. Some tests that you may consider doing are:

- LBT Test (Lactulose Breath Test) to diagnose for SIBO

- IGG Food Sensitivity Test to identify which foods may be causing a response that could have been missed on a food allergy test

- OAT (Organic Acid Test) to check for vitamin and mineral deficiencies that are coming from lack of absorption

- Stool Test to check the balance of good and bad gut bacteria in your digestive tract

Once you have identified the details of your gut issues, you can create a more specific plan, but there are enough commonalities to where you can start working on relief immediately. Many people who work out know the importance of L-glutamine for the recovery of muscles. For similar reasons, it is incredibly beneficial in healing the stomach lining. It is the fuel source for the cells within your small intestine and helps with the food sensitivity response. It is challenging to get enough L-glutamine through diet sources like meats, dairy, beans, raw spinach, red cabbage, and parsley. Due to that lack of availability from natural sources, it is a needed nutritional supplement. It also happens to be incredibly cost-effective. I recommend about five grams of L-glutamine supplement twice daily. Because it has no flavor, I just throw it in my gallon of water and drink it throughout the day.

The next supplement that is important for all types of gut issues is one for digestive support, specifically digestive enzymes. Often, food travels through our body, and we are not able to gain all the positive effects of it. Our digestive tract is not breaking the food down fast enough for it to be absorbed into our cells. Digestive enzymes help the gut not work as hard. They will create quick symptom relief if you struggle with acid reflux, gassiness, bloating, malabsorption, or stool problems.

Getting rid of gluten for a few months is another thing you can do to aid gut recovery. We have done so many artificial things to our wheat that is now packed with gluten. You must be careful as gluten sneaks into many different foods besides wheat products; it acts as a filler and binding agent within many processed foods. It is estimated that gluten is responsible for over 55 diseases and a trigger for many others.

Bone broth and collagen peptide protein are another amazing group of products that can completely transform your health by aiding your gut. They provide vital amino acids like glycine, glutamine, and proline that will drastically help in recovery. Also, the collagen found within them will be awesome for your skin and hair. Most importantly, it acts as a gut sealer. Because if your gut is leaking, it makes sense to seal it, right? The products also give you amazing minerals like calcium, magnesium, phosphorus, sulfur, and silicone in an easy to absorb form.

Fermented vegetables and dairy are also great sources of relief for digestive issues because they help to get more healthy gut bacteria into our system. Fermented veggies are also easier to digest than raw ones, giving your body a lot of nutrients without having to work extra hard. Two of the most common ones are kimchi and sauerkraut, but there are other, drinkable options out there, like kombucha. With dairy, your go-to should be kefir as it is full of fantastic bacteria and helps with dairy tolerance. Yogurt is awesome, too; remember to go for the all-natural kind and none of that low or non-fat stuff you find all over grocery store shelves.

There are many solutions out there that will work wonders for you, but it is not always easy to commit to. Do you know why it is tough to get people to make the changes in order to recover their gut health? People have forgotten what good feels like and do not have a good comparison to work from. You have been this way for many years. The best thing I can tell you is to do a 30-day challenge and pay attention to how you feel during the day. With awareness, you will see what your body should feel like, and you will be much more likely to stay with this for the long term. Because it can take up to six months for your gut to be fixed.

PART 3

Nutrition

CHAPTER 15

Forgetting the Foundation Paper Cut

She was doing five group fitness classes, three days of cardio, and an at-home ab workout. This client came to me because she heard that I could help her get the six-pack she had been working so hard for. She was in her mid-40s, and after doing an intake with her, I quickly saw the problem. She was exercising plenty, but her nutrition was off. She was under a lot of stress and not dealing with it well. To help manage symptoms of high stress, she would drink almost on a nightly basis. She was a busy professional and would often skip meals because of the demand on her time. The issue, as most commonly is the case, was that she was not regulating her blood sugar, and due to that, her body was not burning fat well. By trying to solve all her health issues by exercising more, my client was a typical case I would run into. Although I am an advocate for creating a caloric deficit for the day by increasing output, I know that you cannot out-train a poor diet. This wrong mindset is a massive paper cut that many people make. They kill themselves in the gym but do not do the right thing in the kitchen. Without nutrition, there is no health as it is the foundation for EVERYTHING!

Most people overcomplicate nutrition. My approach with my clients has always been to use the 80/20 approach. It means that 80 percent of the time, we are following good habits, and the other 20 percent of the time, we are operating with more nutritional freedom. If someone tries to always be perfect, they end up never being perfect. We must give some wiggle room within the plan to be able to make it a lifestyle rather than a last-minute study session. A diet is like cramming for a test, you don't necessarily learn and are not able to apply the knowledge.

There are some cautions we must consider with the 80/20 approach. We have to be realistic with what that 20 percent looks like. Say you want to have 80 percent of your meals consist of good quality choices, and for the other 20 percent of your meals, you will have the freedom to eat what you want. To make this happen, you must pay attention to frequency and quantity. That means that if you give yourself one meal a day to cheat with, you would be required to have four quality meals. Also, the number of calories you ingest (no need to be precise, just estimate) has to match that formula. Say you were grazing all day with quality food and came home starving. You may have eaten only 1/3 of your daily needed intake, but this deficit does not mean you get to make it up with poor quality, high caloric foods like potato chips and cookies. In this case, you need to make sure that you are eating four meals that are about 80 percent of your daily needed calories and then just getting the other 20 percent with bad choices.

Some will try to say that they will be good all week and then have a cheat day. Well, what often happens and shows up as many of the paper cuts that bring us down is, once again, the uneven spread in caloric intake. Good food is filling, so for six days, if you ate well, you probably kept your calories in a moderate place. Bad foods do not signal satiety to the brain as quality foods do. That is why you tend to overconsume calories on a bad day. The same rule must apply in that, if you take one day to cheat, you cannot eat more calories on that day than you would on other days. That is not an easy task. For this and other reasons, I am not a fan of cheat days, but am perfectly ok with cheat meals if you meet the above-mentioned guidelines.

The other problem we run into with a full cheat day is how hard it is to get back to normal eating. Our mindset gets thrown out of alignment, and that creates massive cravings the following day which make it so much harder to stay disciplined. You may try to justify it to yourself, but in reality, it is not just a discipline issue anymore but a body's demand to get sugar. This happens because, after that day, your body will not be good at regulating blood sugar. I will cover that in much greater detail when we discuss the paper cuts of poor blood sugar regulation later in the book.

There is one caveat to the 80/20 rule. If your digestion is not doing well, you do not get to act on this rule. You won't correct those internal issues if you keep putting in foods that do not belong in your body due to allergies, intolerances, or sensitivities. We often think that it is not a big deal to have a gluten sensitivity and eat a small amount of bread with dinner, but that is most definitely a bad train of thought. When correcting digestion, you need to be committed 100 percent of the time, or you will not get to a place where it is optimized. Think about it as a prison sentence. Your gut will need x amount of time to get better and heal itself. What happens when you try to break out of prison? You get more time added, and if you keep doing it, you may end up with more time on your record than your original sentence. The same things happen in your gut. If you do not stay clean, it is not just a pause and resume type of thing. It is like the time restarts again, and this time, it may be even longer to get there. You need high levels of discipline if you have digestive issues or have things like leaky gut. It means increased intestinal permeability.

To stay disciplined, we need not merely use logic but change our emotional relationship with food. Don't you wish that a time could come where you want the good foods the same as the way you want the bad foods now? Where you look at a menu, and you automatically go for the better choice without giving the poor choice even the slightest consideration? Well, it is possible with proper mind training and awareness. When you start looking at your nutritional intake as not a diet but fuel for your body's performance, it helps you to avoid poor foods and choose the better foods. To begin this shift, you must pay attention to how you feel when you make nutritional choices. It may be useful to start a nutritional journal and not merely record what you ate, but also how you felt afterward. Record things like energy levels, motivation, desire to be around people, feeling of wholeness and fulfillment, satiety, hunger levels, and cravings amongst many other things that you could identify. It is ok to make those bad choices. Eventually, if you do, it will become easy not to want to make them because you will know what great feels like and will not want to compromise that for the temporary pleasure of appeasing a craving.

I do not want you to be like my client. Working out is time-consuming, and it takes us away from other things we love. This fact means that we need to protect our time investment by doing the right thing with our nutrition. You will have ups and downs, but the quality of the food you put into your body needs to be the most important thing you focus on with your health.

CHAPTER 16

Deficiency Paper Cut

I could see the level of frustration on her face when I started questioning her diet. She had been pediatrician for the last 20 years and felt that her knowledge of what was good and what was bad was accurate. I knew that the problem was that the last time she took a nutrition class was over 20 years ago in college. Obviously, nutritional knowledge has shifted a significant amount over that time frame. The things she believed were true did not hold up in the modern age. She was eating clean food, but due to being raised on Indian cuisine, she was consuming more starches compared to other things. Every meal and snack had a significant amount of starchy foods, and even though the quality was good, she was eating way too many carbohydrates per day. She was not aware of this as she had never logged her food. As part of her nutrition coaching, she began a journal and this helped her see what I was seeing.

For this knowledge to bring change, I had to let her get to that realization herself. When we switched out some snacks and modified her sides, her weight started to melt off.

Before we dive into more complex concepts, we need to briefly look at the basics of the food that we eat. Understanding the function and source of the elements in our diet is essential for ensuring we structure our food choices to be in alignment with our individual goals and physiology. When we think about walking into a gym on day one and lifting 300 lbs. overhead, we understand that we need to build our nutritional plan like a good house. It must have a very solid foundation to withstand the storms of life.

Before we start to lay bricks, we must understand how and where to acquire the materials needed. Well, we must follow this same approach in building our nutritional intake. Notice I said nutritional intake, not diet. The reason for this has to do with diets being for the short-term. We are in it for the long term, and you need to learn how to eat well and keep eating that way. Do this not because you want to lose weight, but because it is the best way to optimize your body at all levels, daily.

To begin, let's break down food into two of the most prominent groups there are: micronutrients and macronutrients. Do not let the name fool you as they are both essential. Macronutrients are required in large amounts as they serve as building blocks for energy production and many other aspects of your body. Most foods have each of the three macronutrients in them; they just come in different amounts. Our bodies respond differently to varied daily amounts of each, and they can be used to adjust health, weight, and performance when modified throughout the day. This is one of many reasons why the same diet does not work for everyone as our individual bodies respond differently to the intake of each macronutrient. The main thing to take away here is that none of these three are bad. When eating them in a very disproportionate way, however, it can then become a problem. The nutrition industry makes billions of dollars telling people how these macronutrient ratios are the most important thing out there. I am here to tell you it is not as precise as they say.

The first macronutrient is my favorite: protein. It is derived both from animal and plant sources but is much more concentrated and easily attained through eating meat and fish. Proteins provide us with amino acids, which the body both manufactures and obtains from external sources. When not taken in at the right amount, there are problems that will keep our bodies from being optimized and thriving. Out of the 20 different amino acids, 9 are essential, meaning that our bodies do not produce them on their own. One of the biggest nutritional paper cuts is not eating enough protein every day. There are tales out there that eating too much protein is bad, but it is not scientifically backed. As long as there is not a preexisting kidney condition, science tells us that we are safe to eat large quantities of protein. Some good sources of protein are beans, pulses and legumes, seeds (hemp, chia, flax), unsalted nuts, quinoa, avocado, beets, raw greens (kale, spinach), and obviously meat and fish.

The next macronutrient is fat. For many years, our society was afraid of fat, and we went on low-fat or no fat diets. To make food taste and feel right after taking the fat out, they must add a bunch of artificial stuff, which is never good. Think of your body as the most critical piece of machinery in the world. It will adjust to anything that you do to it to survive. This fact is seen when our bodies shift toward energy conservation when we are not taking in an adequate number of calories daily.

Similarly, our body can adjust to what it uses for a fuel source. We will cover this in greater detail in the metabolism section. You must understand that if you stop eating fat, your body will potentially see it as a less abundant nutrient. Then it will burn less of it throughout the day. The lack of fat burn is not just a problem for weight loss; it causes all sorts of other metabolic disruptions. Fat signals the production of a hormone called leptin, which signals to the brain that we have taken in enough energy. Carbohydrates do not do this. To explain this to my clients, I point out that we can put away half a loaf of bread with some peanut butter and jelly and a glass of milk and not feel full until our belly is bloated. Then, when we try to eat a couple of avocadoes which are 95 percent fat, we lose the desire to keep eating. In this example, you see how leptin works. We will discuss leptin and the other hunger hormone at a later chapter, but the main takeaway here is that fat is our friend. Some examples of healthy fats are almonds, walnuts, seeds (pumpkin, chia), olives, avocados, oils like red palm, grapeseed, olive, avocado, and coconut, as well as fish- and meat-based fats.

The last, and often misrepresented, macronutrient is carbohydrates. The weight loss industry and many 25-year-old Instagram sensations with six-packs have made carbohydrates seem evil. Many say that you are not losing weight just because you smelled a carb last week. This misunderstanding usually stems from trying to explain more complex mechanisms in the body with just macronutrient balance. Carbohydrates, however, are a great and quick form of energy. They are incredibly important for performance and muscle growth due to their impact on insulin. We can survive without them, but why limit our options on what our bodies can have for fuel?

What I teach is that you need to earn your carbohydrates, and I don't mean you earn them only through a grueling one hour workout. Imagine your muscles are like gasoline tanks that hold the carbohydrate fuel for our bodies. Some of it resides in the bloodstream, but our muscles hold the majority of the available energy building blocks. If your gas tank is full in your car, would you go and add more gas into the tank? No, you would not. Why? Because it would overflow due to the storage limit having been reached. The same thing happens in your body, and it is one of the biggest paper cuts to our system.

If you have not depleted the stored fuel through a workout or a prolonged time without having any fuel, you should not add more into the system. The way that overflow shows up in our body has to do with what our body does with energy. If our system sees that we have an overabundance of energy that it cannot readily use, it will store it in a different form for later use. Many of us, or I should say most of us, are not fans of this long-term storage of energy as it equals body fat. Now, if we have used up the fuel in our muscles and we ingest carbohydrates, it is a good thing as it fills up our storage tanks. It also helps with many other bodily functions, one of which is muscle building. We will discuss these concepts in much greater detail when we talk about the importance of blood sugar regulation in optimizing our mental and physical performance. Some examples of great carbohydrate options would be vegetables, even starchy ones, and low glycemic fruit like berries, pomegranate, apricot, kiwi, and grapefruit. Also, some complex grains like buckwheat and quinoa.

The second category of building blocks we must understand are micronutrients, which we commonly refer to as vitamins and minerals. The amount of these nutrients we intake may be minimal, typically under 100 milligrams daily, in comparison to the many grams of daily macronutrients. The vitality to our cellular health is hugely dependent on getting these micronutrients into our body. I am sure you can understand the paper cut problem here. Because the overall amounts are so low, the deficiencies and symptoms do not show up overnight. It is not until repeated micronutrient paper cuts occur that you start to see signs of ill effects, possibly not until years down the road. Thirteen elements originate from Earth's soil and are not made by your body. Plants are the primary source of nutrients for us. Many years ago, I went to a presentation by a famous naturopath. He discussed how our micronutrient deficiencies cause many adverse side effects. If we understood this better in our Western medicine, we could help alleviate the many side effects that come from some of the drugs that doctors prescribe regularly. I had my mind blown when he listed some of the conventional medicines we take for heartburn, statins, and blood pressure and some of the most common side effects. Then he wrote down what micronutrients those medications deplete in our body. Then he followed up with the side effects of that micronutrient depletion, and sure enough, they matched up. It is very important for people to know what role micronutrients play in our body. Although we only need a small amount, they are mighty in power and need to be in abundance.

Micronutrients include such minerals as fluoride, selenium, sodium, iodine, copper, and zinc. They also include vitamins such as vitamin C, A, D, E, and K, as well as the B-complex vitamins. They are necessary for the healthy function of all your body's systems, from bone growth to brain function.

Some of the important functions of individual micronutrients include how sodium maintains the water balance in our system that can affect blood pressure. We need a certain amount of water in our bloodstream to keep a normal blood pressure. Too much of it leads to high blood pressure, and too little of it means getting lightheaded when we stand up. Sodium also plays a massive role in our bodies' pH balance, which is extremely vital to our wellbeing.

Manganese promotes bone formation, energy production, and helps our system to break down the macronutrients that we discussed earlier. You can understand how something that helps to break down the materials needed to produce energy is an important part of our whole operation.

Magnesium deficiency is one of the most significant shortages we see in the U.S. Research estimates that 85 percent of Americans are deficient in magnesium. This fact is scary because magnesium plays a role in over 300 different functions in the body. It helps your heart maintain its normal rhythm. It helps your body convert glucose into energy. It is necessary for the metabolization of two micronutrients, calcium and vitamin C. Magnesium is often depleted during times of high stress or physical activity and a deficiency can show up in symptoms like restless legs, Charley horses/cramps, and muscle spasms. A few years back, before I understood the role of magnesium in my body, I had restless legs syndrome. I would go to bed and rub my feet together as I laid there trying to get comfortable. I do not use lotion, so the skin would make a rough sound due to the friction, and this was not something my wife enjoyed hearing at night. She already had sleep issues (we fixed them later), and this was not helping. On top of drinking more of my green smoothies, I started to take Cal/Mag at night for about two weeks, at 300 mg per day. Then I started doing the second dose in the morning until my symptoms disappeared, and I returned to a maintenance dosage. Magnesium is one of the four supplements I recommend everyone in the world take if their doctor permits it. It is a natural diuretic, so taking too much at once can be a problem with bathroom time. Build up slowly and see how your body responds as you add more and more into your day.

Iron helps your body produce red blood cells and lymphocytes. It also plays a big role in energy production. It controls oxygen deliverability within the cells and can make people feel very out of shape when it is deficient. I once had a very fit client who suddenly started having a lot of fatigue. When she worked out, she could only do maybe half of what she used to, and we investigated so many different things to try to find the answer. We looked at hormones, digestion, and stress response. Finally, when she did a comprehensive lab panel, we uncovered a significant iron deficiency, and she started feeling so much better after supplementation began. However, iron can be toxic, and you should only supplement with it under professional supervision with lab testing.

Iodine helps thyroid gland development and function. It helps your body break down fats, which we all know is important, and it promotes energy production and growth. Many people look to nutrition to lose weight or maintain their goal weight. Something like an iodine deficiency can throw the entire plan off the rail because of the thyroid slowing down and the metabolism becoming less efficient.

I am not going to be able to cover all the problems we may face when our micronutrients are not in balance. However, I want you to understand the impact that this deficiency can have so the next time you have a symptom of something, you don't just grab a pill to cover it up. Ask better questions to uncover what the source of the problem could be and possibly find out the deficiency that may be causing it. This way, you can supplement or eat the right foods to correct it at the root.

CHAPTER 17

Breakfast Paper Cut

Many people tend to simplify things and put the body into a linear functioning system, but that kind of approach is a mistake. Our body is incredibly complex. We must expand our knowledge base just a bit to understand why some common misconceptions can be the paper cuts that are leading to our nutritional downfall. One of these is the idea that, since carbohydrates are bad for you, you should eat them early in the day. You think that your body will not store the carbs as fat because you will burn them up with your daily activity. There is some truth to this, but when we are eating, what are we ultimately after? Are we after burning something up and losing weight, or are we after fueling our system to optimize all our functions, including weight management? I hope that you are beginning to accept that it is the latter of the two. If approached correctly, the first will happen through the focus on the second but not the other way around.

There are many applications to nutrient timing. Here I want to dive into just a few examples so you can begin to see the paper cuts that happen from eating at specific times versus alternative options. This understanding is my continual focus for you to optimize your body, mind, and spirit.

I once had a client who was a nuclear medicine nurse and worked in a very stressful environment. She often covered the typical 12 plus hour shift that often included overnights. She came to me to lose a lot of weight. She had been struggling due to having thyroid cancer and the subsequent tumor removal. Her life stress alone was enough to overwhelm anyone. On top of that, to keep the cancer away, her doctors used high dosages of medication to keep her thyroid in a hyper state. This state was a constant cause of stress.

When she first started to work out, she could not make it through 15 minutes of exercise without becoming extremely tired and light-headed. The stress that she had been through and the constant fluctuations of blood sugar made her very hypoglycemic. If you are not familiar with the term, it means that her body would burn through her carbohydrate storage and have no available fuel to utilize within the workout. Part of the problem was that her body was not good at accessing fat for fuel due to being so dependent on carbohydrates. She thought that she needed to eat a lot of carbs to give her body fuel, but I had her do something a bit different. She started eating very complex carbs—not too many of them. I also had her eat a lot more fats and proteins before working out so her blood sugar would be more stable. Sure enough, each workout extended in duration, and she was able to maintain a higher and higher intensity. I was, and am still, so proud of her for the achievements that she made. Although she faced difficulties, through nutrient timing corrections she lost 60 lbs. in about nine months. This accomplishment came after she could not lose a pound for six months while following the standard practices on her own.

Why was her body able to make such positive changes if she was not loading up on carbohydrates for fuel before a workout? Your body is the most efficient piece of machinery in the world. It will adjust to anything that you may do to it. Those adaptations are meant for survival and if implemented properly, can be positive and, if not, can be very harmful. If you give your system one particular fuel in abundance, it will learn to consume a large portion of needed energy from that fuel. If the fuel source shifts, consumption will switch more toward the new source. Her body became less dependent on blood sugar for fuel and was able to utilize her fat storages. This increase gave her long-lasting energy for her job and workouts. I will cover why this happened more in the metabolism chapter. I want you to know that I did not stop her from eating carbohydrates. We simply shifted the timing of intake. It is not easy at first as the body goes through a transitionary period. During this time, you may feel a bit low, but within a few days, you will notice the shift beginning to happen. Your body starts to access more and more energy from fat in the process of preserving the limited blood sugar and keeping a more consistent energy level, not just in a workout but throughout the day.

All of this has to do with what happens on a cellular level when we eat certain foods. We will cover this by looking at why breakfast is so crucial for your body. Many people argue about the importance of meals. Before we start to argue, let's establish the fact that all meals are important. I am here to discuss breakfast for health purposes, with the specific point of optimal nutrient timing. Breakfast starts our pattern of blood sugar regulation for the day, which sets our hunger levels, food cravings, energy, and even behavioral responses. Have you heard the saying "eat breakfast like a king, lunch like a prince, and dinner like a peasant"? It is referring to structuring your meals backward, with the largest occurring in the morning. In case by case scenarios, this application can be adjusted based on the lifestyle of the individual. I am trying to show you some basics that will change your life, and in due time, you can add on to this knowledge.

Let's first examine the typical breakfast that we have conditioned ourselves to eat. A light breakfast is what I hear many of you do. You eat things like cereal, toast, or waffles. Once again, I am not here to argue the different types of choices within those categories as some are better than others. The bread that has a lot of fiber in it is better than regular white bread, and granola cereal is better than cheap, sweet cereal. What I want you to look at here is the complexity of the food you are eating. If it already has been processed, it makes it easier to digest. Taking away that extra work with digestion creates a large amount of quick energy, as opposed to something that your body has to work to break down. Compare an English muffin to a sweet potato. The sweet potato will take much longer to break down. It is full of fiber, so it will not create a big blood sugar spike unlike the English muffin. So, if we start with simple carbohydrates in the morning, we will create an overburn of blood sugar as your body tries to get rid of the excess quickly. This shift in energy consumption means that you will not be burning fat as well.

You will consume your limited blood sugar to a point where, before the next meal occurs, you will get hungry. Other symptoms include an energy drop and a loss of focus. This scenario is probably the worst one of the three that I am covering, even though you are taking in food. The reason is that, typically, it is a low number of calories, and it sends your body on a blood sugar rollercoaster throughout the day, causing lousy food choices, feelings of being hangry, and many other possible side effects.

The next scenario has you skipping breakfast altogether. This case is not optimal either but can be used as a tool if you control other components of your diet and physiology. Sleeping well plays a significant role in being able to skip breakfast and not have negative ramifications from it. Why? When you do not sleep well, you do not regulate your blood sugar well. Also, you do not control your hunger well. This problem makes it much more critical to manage those to components through breakfast. In the case of skipping breakfast, you do not start with a big blood sugar spike from eating simple carbohydrates. As you go about your day, your blood sugar continues to fall. It falls until you ingest something to bring it back up.

Ability to skip breakfast also depends on your energy expenditure in the morning and how vital your body/brain performance and focus are during that time. If you skip breakfast, then lunch becomes the next most important thing out there, and you need to follow a similar guideline as you do with a good breakfast. You probably have heard about intermittent fasting, but that is not a sustainable way of eating. I am here to teach you a nutritional plan designed to fuel your body, lose weight, and perform. Anyone can maintain the plan for the long-term because it is not a diet. It does not deprive you of things and restrict your life to the point of relapse. What I teach is a set of general parameters that you can adjust based on your lifestyle and preference.

Now, I will tell you to follow these guidelines for the optimal breakfast: start with just fat and protein and minimize carbs to low glycemic carbohydrates that do not spike blood sugar too much or avoid them altogether. Remember, you must have used up the stored carbohydrates before you add more to your body. We do not want to convert that excess into the complex energy storage called fat. Second, try to make it at least 1/3 of your daily calories. There is no need to count daily, but you should have an idea of what your overall intake is. We are creatures of habit and eat similar things every day so ballparking will be just beautiful.

This way of eating gives your body complex fuels that it can use because you already have stored blood sugar in your muscles. It gives you a great start on your caloric intake, and it ensures you are not coming home hungry and needing to grab the first simple snack you see in the cupboard.

Psychologically, when we start our day well, we want to keep the good streak going. We typically make much better nutritional choices, as well as many other choices for the day due to the excellent start. There is a famous video out there with an admiral discussing how to be successful in life. He talks about if you want to win your day, make your bed. That pattern will create a positive ripple effect for the rest of your day. I say if you want to win your day, master your breakfast.

The cool thing about this approach is that you do not need to take my word for it. I want you to run a simple experiment on yourself, and within a day you will be able to notice a difference.

Throughout this book, I want to influence you to make better life choices to stop the thousands of daily paper cuts that could be happening. To make this influence, I need to tell you how to do it, but probably more important than that, I need to show you why it is worth it. The "worth it" component comes from observing the way you feel and experience daily life due to those choices. As you notice the positive feeling, you will establish a better association with the right decisions. This awareness eventually leads to building a habit instead of something you disciplined yourself to do temporarily.

So, one day wake up and have a toast, cereal, and banana type breakfast. Notice how your hunger is by lunch. Notice how your energy and focus are mid-afternoon. Pay attention to the food choices, especially at dinner, that you make. The next day, load up with a big meal and make it fat- and protein-based. My favorite way is with nuts and meats. Yes, this means you have to change how you look at breakfast. I follow this routine because of how it makes my body and brain ready for the day. I cook a ton of meat for dinner and have some leftover with a cup of nuts for breakfast. I do the leftover trick if I do not want to make some fresh steak, bacon, or salmon in the morning.

These two approaches will show you the opposite ends of the spectrum and motivate you directly through observation of the self. Later, you may find a place somewhere in the middle and eat scrambled eggs with some spinach and strawberries on the side for example. Do not feel like you must be boring at breakfast as the principles are intentionally broad to allow for your lifestyle and creativity to individualize the plan.

I hope, through this nutritional shift, you can see how little choices, like when we eat certain foods, can create massive repeated paper cuts on your health and performance.

CHAPTER 18

Calorie Fallacy Paper Cut

One of my hardest working clients was not able to lose weight because of an HCG diet that screwed up her hormones and her metabolism. It is a popular diet that seemed to work for others, so she jumped in headfirst and was fully committed. Just like many in her situation, she began to lose weight. Excited, she dutifully followed the regimented diet that required her to consume HCG, a drug designed to help with women's fertility, and limit fat intake to a minimum. These dieters report that HCG reduces their appetite and gives them the energy that allows them to sustain a caloric intake of no more than 500 calories per day. Her results began to slow, but she remained committed until she no longer saw anything on the scale changing. Frustrated, she came off the diet, and like many others who quit, she binged on all the foods she had deprived herself from eating. Her weight ballooned, and she was much heavier than when she started. It was not surprising for me because I know that the FDA clearly states that HCG is not for weight loss.

The caloric restriction was only able to fool the body so much. Our bodies adjust to the low intake and lower our metabolisms to survive. The body lowers some of its functions to require less calories for fuel. This adaptation leads me to the next set of paper cuts made by people trying to get healthy through their diet. Her caloric restriction was extreme, but it does not take much to disrupt our metabolisms over a long time. This kind of disruption occurs when people start counting calories, which often leads to not eating enough. It is not a permanent disruption as research says that metabolic damage does not happen from dieting. The problem is that recovery is difficult following a significant caloric deficit period. I will talk about this in the chapter focusing on weight on the scale, but the muscle loss is what creates the big problem.

We are not all the same when it comes to size and metabolism. We understand this, yet somehow women have the magical 1,200–1,500 number of calories they are permitted to eat in a day, and men have 1,800–2,000. I know women who eat over 3,000 calories per day, and their performance and body shape would be desired by many. This information is to illustrate my point. Caloric counting creates so many unnecessary steps and the cons outweigh the pros. Now, let me be clear that I am not advocating against journaling food or paying attention to what we eat. You should remember quality is what comes first. We must apply the next steps as we master the previous and determine the necessary follow-up based on the size of the goal that you are trying to accomplish. I am against the need to count calories and the lack of proper application that people tend to create. If you are struggling with eating clean and natural food, you need to focus on establishing consistency there before ever counting calories. The only time I would take that approach is if I was prepping a competitor for a bodybuilding show or an athlete for very high-level performance.

The other problem with counting calories is that the numbers you find on labels are estimates and not exact. In a study where different foods were measured by the number of calories they have, there was a big discrepancy found between all the different readings. The FDA allows for up to 20 percent error on labels. So, let's think about this. Many people are stressing about eating half of a nut to make sure they get enough fat, yet the measurement already could be off. Why bother trying to get something exactly perfect when there is no control over that 20 percent variance?

The other reason why calorie counting is not necessary and more of a nuisance than an advantage is that not all foods are equal. Well, of course, Anton, many of you will say, but what I am talking about is absorption rates. You will hear people say that you are what you eat, and I will always correct them and say you are what you absorb. There are two components that we must look at here. First, the health of your digestive system varies. Depending on how well you are doing, it changes how much of the same nutrient you can absorb on any given day. If you do not absorb something into your bloodstream, then it is not going to count as calories going into your body. That food passes through and goes out with the waste. The other, and even a bigger, component is that not all foods are absorbed equally. Most people know that a gram of carbohydrate and protein produce four calories each and a gram of fat produces nine calories. What most people do not know is that there is still a variance between what percentage of that food will be absorbed. For example, when you eat an almond, a healthy digestive system will typically absorb about 68 percent of that nut. When we compare it to a different member of the nut family, like a pistachio, then we see that 95 percent of it is absorbed.

Everything I just described has to do with the equation of the energy balance. It is true that you must eat less than you burn to lose weight or eat more than you burn to gain weight, but is not as simple as that. Why is it inaccurate? There are so many factors that are left out as part of this equation. Both the calories in and calories out components need to be expanded a lot more to make the equation more accurate. Even then, it is nearly impossible to make precise calculations to justify the work of counting everything. Factors influencing calories in: the accuracy of measuring the calories within the food, the ability to absorb the food, and the physiological factors of the individual body like gut health and bacteria balance. Factors influencing calories out: energy burned at rest, energy burned through exercise, energy consumed through non-exercise activity, and energy burned by metabolizing food.

The other struggle with this equation is how to measure calorie expenditure for the day. RMR is a huge component, and there is a lot of variance from person to person which makes this part of the inaccuracy of the equation. As I mentioned in Chapter Nine, RMR is the number of calories you consume if you laid in bed and did absolutely no movement all day long. For example, I am 195 lbs., and most formulas would have my resting metabolism at about 2,000 calories. I have had it measured many times with tools like oxygen measurement, and it comes in around 2,400 calories in reality. I could be spending all this time on logging and counting everything without ever realizing that my body burns 400 more calories per day than I thought. Big error yet again! People can be the same weight, height, and age, but based on their metabolism and oxygen efficiency, they can burn a very different number of calories. I have seen this variance measured at over 550 calories per day when I was a metabolic coach.

The next component that makes measuring calories unhelpful is the thermic effect of eating. It means that when you eat certain foods, your body creates heat, and that utilizes some of that energy.

Have you ever had "meat sweats"? They are a perfect example of how that phenomenon works in application. How in the world are you going to measure this to keep your energy equation accurate?

Then comes the calculation of your physical activity. Just like with resting metabolism, there is a significant variance in active metabolism from person to person even if they are the same age, height, and weight. How can someone accurately count what they burn per day with their activity? Step counters are just an estimation and have a large amount of error.

Finally, your non-exercise activities. Think about it, even as you sit in a chair, how many small movements do you do daily? How does a day of sitting compare to a day of meetings or to a day of presentations? There is a large degree of variance yet again, and it makes it nearly impossible to count caloric expenditure over that time.

Ultimately, what is the point that I am making here? Many health gurus would have you believe in the need for calorie counting and tracking, yet with this many inaccuracies present, why would you spend the time doing it? However, there is something great about tracking calories. It is not a perfect measurement of everything, but the awareness you get from seeing what and how much you have eaten is beneficial. There is no need to measure calories exactly when you have a food journal, it is just so you are aware of what you eat in a day or week.

So, to save time and not place extra stress on you by counting all your calories, I want you to estimate. To do this, I use the system I was taught when I received my Precision Nutrition certifications. It all comes from estimating by using your hand as it makes the perfect tool. Your hand is proportionate to your body, its size does not change, and it is always with you.

Women and men have some variance due to differences in size and metabolism, and they often use their bodies in different ways. Remember that this is an estimation for the average population. If you are an athlete or do things on a higher level, you may need to be more precise.

Starting with fats, a man should have about two thumb-sized portions, and a woman should have one thumb-sized portion. For carbohydrates, a man should have about a two cupped hands portion, and a woman should have one cupped hand. When it comes to proteins, a man should eat two palm-sized portions, and a woman should eat one palm. Last but not least are your veggies, and a man should eat two fist-sized portions while a woman needs one

So, to summarize what I have outlined for you, I want you to realize that calorie counts are imprecise. For different reasons, we don't absorb all the foods we consume and have a hard time counting the calories we expend. It means that calorie counting is just an unnecessary stress that is not worth the work put in. Why are so many people doing it then? Because, out of calorie counting comes a hyper-awareness of what we eat. There is portion control built into your meals, and the process often pushes you to prep meals and to have great food around versus having to go for nutrient poor snacks. It supports food journaling to see how each day and week went. All of these are great tools when implemented in the right order, but they do not require counting calories to be successful.

CHAPTER 19

Supplement Paper Cut

Can I eat natural foods and get enough nutrients that way? If I take supplements, can I get away with not eating vegetables? Those are the two extremes I see when it comes to supplements. The former is thinking that we can always get enough from Mother Nature as long as we eat clean. The latter is thinking that we can do whatever we want because we have this invisible shield of supplements that will protect us from the side effects of the harmful things we put into our bodies. Neither is right.

Starting with natural food is always the right thing to do. Unfortunately, due to our changing environment, we no longer have the things that Mother Nature provides in abundance. When we look at this fact, we must look at our soil. If you compare fruits and vegetables grown in a very commercialized country, like the U.S., to a country that is less developed, you will notice a difference. The produce looks and tastes very different. The taste is much better in those less commercialized countries due to the farming practices and, ultimately, the soil they are grown in. The soil in much of the world has been stripped of very important micronutrients. When the nutrients are not there in quantities needed, we must find alternative ways to get them. This deficiency is why multivitamins are imperative for every single person in the developed world. Take them with meals to ensure they do not upset your stomach, and try to find them with a GMP label, which stands for Good Manufacturing Practices. It gives you the peace of mind that the vitamin is a quality product as there are a lot of bad ones out there due to the FDA not regulating supplements. Soil is supposed to have more than 20 minerals in it, but most farmers just fertilize with anywhere from four to six minerals because that is enough to make produce. Just because large quantities of produce are yielded does not mean they have everything your body needs.

About 65–85 percent of the population in the U.S. is deficient in magnesium, which plays a role in over 300 different bodily functions and why we must get it as a regular supplement. Now, here is where you have an option. You can get magnesium from green leafy veggies or choose to supplement in one of the forms magnesium is offered. In my experience, it is best absorbed through the skin and my clients use magnesium cream under their knees and in the crook of their arm. Also, an excellent way to get it in is through Epsom salt baths. Floatation therapy is a very concentrated form of these baths and has many more positive benefits than just magnesium replenishment. My wife is shy and not a big fan of getting massages because she does not like being touched by strangers. We found that when she goes to the float spas, she gets the same relief and feels just as relaxed, if not more so, than she did after a massage. Try this out by looking up floatation therapy in your area.

Another nutrient that has become more important now than before are omega-3 fatty acids. We used to be able to eat a couple servings of salmon a week and get enough, but unfortunately, now we need to get a lot more than that. Our fish supply in the world has become very polluted, and I caution my clients with their fish choices. When it comes to maintaining a good balance of omega-3 in our body, many people rely on fish oil. I am a big believer in supplementing with omega-3s even if you eat fish. I have had clients take as much as one gram per percent of their body fat when they were aggressively going after weight loss. Typically, I have people take between 4–12 grams. It all depends on the lifestyle and nutritional habits of the individual. You may ask why we need this much, and the answer has to do with how our diets has shifted. Because people eat a lot more grains and processed foods, we are getting more omega-6 content. We only need around a three-to-one ratio of omega-6 to omega-3. In our standard diet, it is estimated that the ratio has skyrocketed to about 16-to-1, which is why we need a lot more omega-3s as a supplement to bring the rate back to a proper alignment. The other reason we need more omega-3s is because our exposure to pollutants and stress has drastically increased, and it has anti-inflammatory properties. Omega-3s have many more positive effects. On top of assisting with weight loss through blood sugar regulation, fish oil in particular helps improve cognition, skin, and hair. Given all that information, it is silly to keep making the paper cut of not getting omega-3s into your body.

Now, there are also many supplements out there that we may need based on individual deficiencies. Due to our environmental factors, the three I already outlined should be taken by every person regardless of goal and current state of nutrition. Next, I will show you some of the popular supplements people take for different reasons.

The first supplement is protein, and the most common form is whey. I see so many people make a paper cut here without ever realizing they are causing harm. I had a client who was determined to get better after she found out she had a dairy sensitivity. She thoroughly cleaned out her diet and initially dropped some weight. All of a sudden, she started feeling sick to her stomach. We thought about everything, and then I found out that she had switched proteins from the collagen protein I had her on to a popular whey protein. Well, there was the problem as the whey comes from milk. The minute we switched her back, she began to feel better and began to lose weight again. So, make sure you understand that there are different types of protein. If dairy is a problem, you may need to take a collagen protein made from cowhide or use a plant-based formula. With a plant-based formula, you may run into digestive issues if you are sensitive to peas; most of the vegan proteins use it as one of the bases.

The other supplement people rely on is a greens supplement to boost their antioxidants and get all the needed nutrients into their body. For this one, my general rule of thumb is that if you eat at least 12 servings of fruits and veggies daily, with veggies being 9 of those servings, you do not need it. The further you are from that number, the more the greens supplement may be required. It is very tasty and easy to add to shakes.

Another supplement that I am a massive fan of and personally use is tyrosine, which is useful for people under chronic stress. It helps to reduce central nervous system fatigue and symptoms of your sympathetic nervous system, the fight or flight response, from overacting during moments of high pressure, workouts, and general life stress.

Let's move on to your favorite supplement: caffeine. It has been demonized by our society, but it is not a bad thing. When used in proper timing, amount, and by the right demographic, it is amazing. The problem is that there is a catch-22. The more you need it for energy, the less you should have as it is a stimulant and you become burned out trying to push your body to the limit. When I coach clients through quitting caffeine, I explain it like a tired runner that has been running behind them for a long time. When they take caffeine, you run up to them and hit them in the back, giving them a jolt momentarily. Ultimately, they will break down their body down the road from the abuse and overreaching for performance.

There are too many supplements for me to explain them all. However, I want you to know there are supplements to help you regulate hormones naturally, help you sleep, and even help you build lean body mass. Regardless of which supplements you consider, you cannot just take them without changing the habits that brought you to the spot you are. Take them while improving your habits to help optimize your body. Which brings me to the other group of people who take supplements. Go to www.ProspectiveForce.com/10percentFITTER and you can get a 25 percent off deal for supplements that I use with our clients.

This group is the one who throws money at the wall and sees what sticks. What I mean by that is when people think they can live however they want because they are supplementing their diet. They eat poorly thinking that if they are taking vitamins, they are fine. That is not the way it works, and you must remember that the word is supplement, not replacement. It is meant to augment our natural intake, not act as something that can completely replace it. So do not think that by taking supplements, you do not have to pay attention to your stress, digestion, and eating habits.

CHAPTER 20

Scared of Fat Paper Cut

As I write this, fewer people believe that eating fat makes you fat than when I started health coaching over a decade ago. But when I look at our yogurt section in the grocery store and see that 90 percent of the options are still saying no fat or low-fat, I feel compelled to cover this. I want to make sure that everyone stops believing this fallacy.

Years ago, I was taught a lesson by my doctor, who was brilliant in naturopathic medicine. He said, "Anton, when you hear the words low-fat or no fat, think of words chemical shit storm." Then he would go on to explain that fat provides a lot of the substance of the food. When it is taken out, other things have to be put in so the food's taste and texture are as similar to the original as possible. These chemicals are not naturally made and do not belong in our body. This switch is primarily targeting the calorie counting population because by taking out the fat, the most calorie-dense macro-nutrient, the total calories of the product are significantly reduced. Now that trade-off is not a positive one as the chemical damage to our cellular health overwhelms the positive effect of fewer calories. It may work on the short-term, but in the long term, it will wreak havoc on your body and create hormonal problems.

The other myth that drives low-fat diets is the fear of cholesterol. Many people still avoid saturated fat, even if it is natural and comes from grass-fed sources. It is due to their doctors telling them that if they eat it, their cholesterol numbers are going to go up. Red meat and eggs are common enemies of these practices. This belief came from a research study conducted in the 1960s. The research did not show a direct correlation, and then for 50 plus years, we believed something that was not true. Cholesterol does matter, don't get me wrong. There is a 500 percent increase in the chance of death when someone goes from 200 mg/dl to 260 mg/dl. These numbers represent the total cholesterol quantity to which your doctor will typically refer. There are also studies showing that low levels of cholesterol may contribute to depression. So, there is a sweet spot for each type of cholesterol.

As you may already know, HDL cholesterol is considered good, and LDL cholesterol can be harmful if it is too high. However, there is more to say about LDL cholesterol because there is a more positive form of it called particle A. It is a large particle and does not cause plaque in the arteries. The bad version of LDL cholesterol is known as particle B, which is small and can cause plaque in the arteries. So, don't assume that always having a high LDL number is a horrible thing. There are proper ratios to all of this, and if you think you have a problem with cholesterol, make sure you can do the NMR (Nuclear Magnetic Resonance) LipoProfile. The NMR is a cholesterol test which provides more information than a standard lipid panel. This test includes measurements for total cholesterol, LDL, HDL, triglycerides, insulin markers, lipoprotein particle number and size, and lipoprotein subfractions. A specialist can interpret the results and help you understand if you should be alarmed or not, and what to do about the cholesterol levels specific to your body.

Fat is not the enemy we have made it out to be because it does not affect cholesterol quite as we had thought. It is more about balance than the total amount consumed. What I mean by that is it is important to eat both saturated and unsaturated fats. Because if you eat too much saturated without enough unsaturated, then you can cause problems with your heart. Also, if you eat a diet high in fat, you do not want to eat a diet high in REFINED carbohydrates. I covered carbohydrates already but remember they must be earned and minimized to a general 80/20 rule. That means 80 percent of them should be unrefined carbohydrates, like quinoa, and 20 percent can be refined, like bread. As far as total fat intake, I suggest having around 30 percent of your total caloric intake coming from fat. Depending on health conditions and goals, that number may go up or down by 10 percent.

Fat is also used for mineral absorption and is vital to hormone production. This connection means that by not getting enough fat in, we can harm many essential processes within our system.

In summary, good quality fat is not the foe that it has been made out to be. In reality, it can be a very great friend.

PART 4

Movement

CHAPTER 21

Cardio Paper Cut

For too many years, the understanding that we need to burn more calories than we consume has driven people toward cardio machines more than anything else in the gym. Yes, even more than booty blast class and Zumba. Ever since I was 11 years old, I have attended the local gym a few times a week. I have noticed that people love to push themselves on cardio, be it with time, intensity, or both, to burn more calories and lose weight faster. But what if we had it wrong all along?

Cardio is defined as exerting yourself above 60–70 percent of your max heart rate output for 20 minutes or greater. Now, don't get me wrong, I am not advocating against cardio. We do need to have proper metabolism, a healthy heart, and burn calories. I am arguing against cardio being the system rather than just a tool and against cardio done with improper intensities and durations based on a person's needs. There are four main paper cuts I want to address here. First, not focusing on adjusting metabolism with cardio. Second, not considering our stress when doing cardio. Third, prioritizing cardio over weight training in limited time scenarios. Finally, not warming up properly before starting the cardio session.

Cardio is a great tool when coupled with the other tools that you have in your health toolbox. They include nutrition, stretching, stress management, weight training, recovery, sleep, and many more. We all know that no matter how much you exercise you get, if you eat poorly, you will eventually end up unhealthy. The same goes for neglecting the other tools. For example, if you only do cardio and never lift weights, you can impose so much stress on your body that you end up gaining belly fat. Yes, too much of a good thing is not a good thing in this situation. Now, when you find the balance between all those tools, life becomes better. With them tailored to your body and lifestyle needs, you become the version of yourself that you were put on this earth to be. Can you imagine the things you can accomplish once you are there?

As I already covered, when desiring change, we need to run to a positive instead of away from a negative. This method applies to the intention behind our positive behaviors, like cardio. We need the right mindset to make the behavior conditioned for us. So, the right mindset for cardio is not to burn calories as that is running from being overweight. Instead, and more accurately, the mindset is to positively impact our metabolism and shift how our body utilizes fuel for energy. Doing cardio to chase weight loss is a big paper cut that people commit because it leads to emotional failure as well as a lack of maximizing what we can get out of it.

We set out to lose weight from cardio, so it is meant to be short-lived and already brings up a negative connotation. Ultimately, it leads to less desire for the action. Yes, people succeed, but it is way less likely until you shift to the mindset of metabolism adjustment. How does the metabolism adjust through cardio? Remember when we talked about our body using a different percentage of fat and different percentage of sugar to fuel itself? The same thing stands true in times of exercise. It has to do with how much oxygen is available and what is the total need for energy for the activity.

There is a sweet spot where the intensity is perfect for fat burn. Also, there is a sweet spot where the intensity is better for teaching your body to pull in more oxygen and strengthen the heart. You can do an active metabolic test, but I typically explain it this way. If you want to burn the most fat while exercising and improve your body's ability to burn fat at rest, do cardio at an intensity where you feel a little out of breath but can hold a conversation freely. If you want to improve your body's oxygen use and heart strength, do cardio at an intensity where you can only say about two to three words per breath. The perfect combination should be both, and I recommend a ratio of four-to-one. This ratio is called interval training and is meant for an average person who wants to be in shape and have a healthy metabolism.

So, how it would break down is that the duration of your cardio workout would be broken up into five minute segments. Each segment would be four minutes of the comfortable conversation pace and one minute of the two to three words per breath pace repeated for the duration of the workout.

To illustrate the point, let's take an hour on the treadmill. I was a Marine many years ago and still have the drill instructor mode that I can turn on to give extra motivation to people. Spit flying, hands waving in your face, and my voice at a decibel level that almost bursts your eardrums. Now, say I became this guy and put you on a treadmill for an hour, "motivating" you the entire time. What will be the outcome? Well, you burned 1,000 calories, you almost died, you do not like me anymore, and you probably do not enjoy cardio. But, you burned 1,000 calories and that's awesome, right? For short-term maybe but remember you do not do cardio just to burn calories but to adapt your metabolism.

We focus on this adjustment because our body consumes so many calories at rest. So, at the intensity you were going during that hour, you only consumed five percent from fat. There was not enough oxygen for the body, and caloric demand was so high that the body had to use a more accessible fuel, like sugar, to produce the energy needed. So, in total, 50 calories of fat were consumed at that intensity. Yes, there is an afterburn, but that's once again just focusing on the caloric burn and not adapting metabolism. That afterburn can be achieved in a fraction of that time as long as we give maximum intensity for the short duration of the interval. For the second scenario, we follow the four-to-one ratio of low intensity to high intensity. You may have burned half the calories in that same hour, but 50 percent came from fat, and your body consumed 250 calories of fat versus just the 50 in the first scenario. The other, and more important, benefit is that we gave your body practice to consume fat at a higher activity level. This adaptation means that, over time, your body improves what percentage of fat it can utilize for fuel. It is incredible what positive impact it has on your resting metabolism and how much it shifts your ability to use fat as a fuel source throughout the day. In summary, it is not just what's right in front of us that is important. We must dig a bit to understand the focus and connect the right actions to it to see success.

Next, the question of duration of the workout, which leads me to the second cardio paper cut of not paying attention to your stress levels. Your body is just a bunch of chemical responses. It does not know if you are exercising or if you are running away from a wild animal. It releases stress chemicals to increase your performance after about 40 minutes of continuous cardio activity. Now, if you are not under chronic stress, this is not a problem as your body recovers after a good rest. However, if your body is already chronically stressed from any of the reasons I'll cover later, this kind of chemical dump will not be beneficial. Hurting your stress response when it is already poor is a lot more costly than what you gain from the positive effects of that cardio session. So, keep your cardio sessions under 40 minutes if you are under chronic stress. For exercise, lean more on weights and circuit-type workouts for maximum efficiency. When you take breaks between sets, your heart rate is not constantly elevated and, in turn, not making your system feel like it is in danger. Circuit training, especially done in a high-intensity format, gives you both the benefits of cardio and weight training if you do not have a lot of time. Now, please do not think this is a quick fix. You have to build up a foundation before getting into workouts like these. I will cover that in a later chapter.

The next paper cut has to do with wanting to do cardio over weight training. Do not get me wrong, I have done over a thousand consultations with new gym members, and I understand why that happens. The answer is one word: intimidation. People are afraid to look stupid or hurt themselves or not get the results that they need from their workouts. They choose the safe and easy route of doing cardio to avoid those fears. It saves you some temporary pain, but in the long run, you are going to miss out on the many benefits of resistance training. I will encourage you to get help if this is a scenario that rings true with you. Invest in a trainer for about three months and watch your life change while you are in the care of their quality hands. Then, use the tools for a lifetime, and when you look at the investment that way, the value skyrockets. Why are weights better than cardio, especially when time is limited? Weights produce more hormonal changes than cardio does, and when there is a spike in our anabolic hormones, we increase our fat burn. High-intensity weight training is the best way to boost these hormones. I will cover more in a future chapter, but you must know that intensity is not always about heart rate. It is all about how much you are exerting yourself compared to your max capability. So, a low repetition and high weight format can also be high intensity and not beat up your body. I have talked about the benefits of raising metabolism through adding muscle mass, but the hormonal impact is even better for you in the long run. I also mentioned that the benefits of cardio could be accomplished with weight training, but the same does not ring true in reverse.

The last papercut I will discuss in this chapter is not getting a proper warm-up prior to the workout. Cardio is great for this for many reasons. It helps you burn more fat during your workout, a fact which I will dive deeper into in the metabolism chapter. Cardio also helps you loosen your muscles and joints. As a low injury risk activity, it helps your body before you start to move in more complex patterns that have a higher chance of causing injury if not properly warmed up. Old ways of warming up included bending over and touching your toes to stretch. We now know, however, that it is not ideal for your muscle to be stretched statically when in a cold state as it can cause injuries and weaken the body before the workout.

In conclusion, cardio is an awesome tool, but it is not as simple as getting on a piece of equipment or being outdoors and going as hard as you can. You now can understand what intensity to use, what duration to go for, and what factors to consider when choosing cardio. Start making these changes and watch the pounds start to fall off, but, most importantly, watch how they stay off because you lost them in the right way.

CHAPTER 22

Stability Paper Cut

I was running across the fitness floor as I typically do when not with a client or doing a consultation. I noticed, out of the corner of my eye, a man waving me over as he took his headphones off. As I looked over at him, I quickly noticed the right side of the body looking like it was causing him pain. It seemed much tighter than the left, and his arm was not as relaxed in the movement. As we began to walk toward each other, he grabbed two different sizes of dumbbells.

Before I was even able to greet him, he said, "Watch this," and grabbed a 35 lb. dumbbell with his left hand and easily lifted it to his side. Then, he grabbed a five lb. dumbbell and failed to repeat the motion on the right side.

As he put the weight down, he said, "Your name is Anton, right? I have seen you training around the gym and have heard many of my gym buddies sing your praises for the things you have done for them. I woke up this way, and it does not hurt, but I cannot raise my right arm to the side to save my life. What do you think happened?"

I walked him over to the stretching table, and we did some manual resistance drills. We worked for a few sessions after that, and he was able to regain normal function as there was no tear present that required surgery or healing. Why did that happen? His body turned off a muscle to avoid injury because he was moving improperly. This injury was due to the poor stability of the shoulder. Instead of using his back to stabilize the shoulders when he bench pressed, his body used the neck.

Doing stability work is not sexy, and it will not make you lose a ton of weight. Without it, however, you have diminished chances of a successful health transformation, and your chances of injury skyrocket. The success rate drops because of many factors. If you do not teach your body to use the muscles in their intended way, your poor movement patterns will lead to unnecessary pain. This inadequacy creates injuries that take you out of training and reverse your strides toward a better metabolism. You exert yourself too much in the beginning and do not build a progressive momentum in your fitness, which leads to a poor relationship with working out.

Think about your joints and tissues that connect everything in the body; this is what you should start working on before beginning an intense exercise regimen. Lifting weights without addressing the stability of the joint is like trying to launch a rocket out of a rowboat in the ocean. Because there is no stable foundation, that rocket will go hard and maybe far, but where it will go is not exactly predictable. Think about the wacky inflatable tube man that you see at car dealerships trying to catch your attention. That is an exaggeration of what you look like when exercising if you do not build up stability in your body.

Now, because of that instability, we get a huge paper cut of pain due to improper movement during the exercise. This outcome comes from joints not moving the way they were intended and the body using muscles not designed for the movement. Your body does this to compensate for the weakness created from lack of stability. This leaves you in a lot more pain than you should be in. Don't get me wrong, a bit of muscle soreness is unavoidable when starting out. However, intense soreness in the wrong area is a sign of doing something wrong. Think about what this does to your mind. Are you more likely to work out when your body is in pain or when you feel good? Are you more likely to stick to working out if you believe in "no pain, no gain" or if you feel amazing after each workout? Well, of course it is the latter, but to do that you must start small, move fast, and think big. Working on little muscles and doing light workouts may seem tedious, but if it leads you to the shape you always dreamed of, it is a sacrifice you must make.

Some muscles are designed more for holding things, and some are more designed to move them. You need to make sure that you pay attention to both, equally. Workouts can become progressively harder and even lead to weight loss when we focus on the holding muscles over time. Yoga is a great example. Yoga gives you more flexibility, helps your stability and mobility, and it also reduces stress. Yoga should be a staple for anyone on a weight loss journey, but as a tool, not as a complete system.

Why? Because yoga is inadequate for weight loss and should be paired with regular weight training for the greatest success.

Often, I hear people say, "I am very flexible and stretch all the time. I do not need to worry about stability workouts." This statement is a big misconception as people think of flexibility as stability and mobility. It is not the same, and we need to understand the difference. Flexibility is just the ability to lengthen a muscle to its most extended form. Stability means holding with control in a specific area. The culmination of the two is mobility, and that is the ability to take a joint through its intended full range of motion with control and in a proper movement pattern. This is why you see so many mobility workout videos popping up. People realize that aging well and being able to live your life into your 80s has to do with how well you move.

Once you understand the importance of a stable foundation, you start to fall in love with your results. It comes not just from the weight coming off your body, but from how you can use your body better. This improvement is where small wins create a ton of motivation. When you look at it from the right perspective, your desire to work out increases, which then leads to more weight loss. It also helps you realize the infinity goal of always improving your ability to do things with your body. It is exciting, fun, and what I attribute to a large portion of my success with my clients as a health coach.

Stability training does not mean you do it once and stop. Your body adapts over time, and you should push it hard to get the proper progression. If not, you tend to create compensation patterns during this time. So, this foundational component should be revisited every three to four months to ensure you rebalance and to realign everything in your body to function as optimally as possible. You must keep building the difficulty of the stability workouts so you keep progressing and challenging your body. Even when they are tougher, these workouts are still a break from the other hard exercises you do.

This practice ensures that you do not come to the point of diminishing results, where you get fewer results even though you are trying more.

When working on stability, you must have the right mindset of chasing proper movement with a slow tempo and full control. It is not about weights. Each repetition could take you as long as 10 seconds to complete and most likely does not require much weight, if any. As you progress, you want to challenge the stability of the environment by making your platform less stable. Initially, you can start by standing on the floor and holding onto something. Then, you can progress to not holding anything. From here, you can move to using a half blue ball, called a BOSU ball, to make the ground more wobbly. There are many apparatuses designed to change the stability of what you are standing on, so play around and keep it fun. From there, you can start adding weights as well.

Stability, flexibility, and mobility may not be the sexy workouts you desire, but they are the ones that will create a foundation that you can build a mountain on, without worrying if everything falls apart because you got hurt.

CHAPTER 23

Workout Paper Cut

Instagram and Facebook are flooded with content claiming to include "The Best Exercise to Burn Fat." You can get six-pack abs in 30 days if you do this one thing. You can lose 21 lbs. in 21 days if you do this other thing. All of these are just gimmicks to get you to click on the post and follow them or buy from them. These are very easy to fall prey to because they play on our incredibly powerful emotions. That is one of the reasons why the health industry is booming with revenue now more than ever, and it is projected to grow exponentially.

I want you to run away from anything that seems like a quick fix as it simply does not work. It may help in the short-term and then cause issues down the road, or it quickly stops working and gets you nowhere close to the promise made. I hope that by reading this book, you are beginning to understand the importance of custom tailored solutions to your health transformation journey. Many factors need to be considered when choosing an exercise program. Some things to look at: your stress levels, your energy levels, your time available, your support system, your financial resources, and your current state of health and fitness, among other things. Why am I mentioning this? Because for each factor there is a different regiment or exercise

I would have you try. I am going to cover some of the best activities that you should do after building up a stable foundation based on what we talked about before.

There are some common concepts that I want to introduce before going over a few staple exercises that can help you. The focus is to not make the paper cut of following gimmicky advice. You want to move large muscle groups to create the best hormonal response and burn the most calories. You also want to have a high-intensity approach that spikes your metabolism. You want to focus on exercise selections that are balanced and are not going to create injuries. To top it off, you want a workout regimen that is hitting on all needed components of fitness. Finally, you should take advice from people who focus on the demographic that you belong to. All exercises are applied differently depending on your actual body.

I do not know how many times I have seen an overweight person trying to lose weight with their trainer motivating them for one more rep with a bicep curl. I want to run up to the trainer and yell at them for wasting the client's time and money, but of course, I bite my tongue. Often, after the session is over, I will pull the trainer aside and ask them what they are thinking and why they chose that exercise selection. Do you want to know the standard answer? They tell me, "Well, I want to make sure we cover all important muscles for the body." Important for what? This lack of awareness is a common mistake, leading to following general workouts instead of programming specific to the goal. For weight loss, doing a bicep curl by itself is one of the biggest time wasters. If someone wants to do bicep curls, they should incorporate them with a more significant movement, like a lunge or a squat. Even though it seems silly, you can train while utilizing larger muscle groups of other movements in the exercise selection. Once you have built your foundation, you want to focus on triple joint exercises. This focus means that you are using three joints at once while moving. Examples include variations of squats, lunges, deadlifts, step-ups, rows, pulls, presses, and many more. Do not waste your time on small muscle movements until you have lost most of the weight, and your goal begins to shift to some other focus.

There was a period in my life where I worked in the same gym for three and a half years. It was a gym where I was part of the grand opening. Before I transferred to another location, there were still quite a few founding members around that I would see five days a week. They would go to the typical group fitness classes. Throughout that period, their physique hardly changed at all. Why did that occur? The answer has to do with one of my favorite things to say to people: 90 percent of the difference occurs in the last 10 percent of your effort. This statement means that when you are doing 10 reps, you must pick a weight that you can barely finish for 10. That last rep is the one that signals your body a need for change as it is slightly outside of your current comfort zone. This signaling increases the hormones that burn fat and create muscle. The people I am talking about were not pushing themselves enough. Their bodies had gotten used to what they were doing and not asking for something outside of their capabilities, so the need for change was not in their system. This failure is why adding progressive intensity into your workouts is so important. It is not always about pushing until failure. If you do, you will crash your system. Instead, strategically pick days or phases that force you to your limit. Just make sure you provide adequate recovery and nutritional support to sustain this.

In exercise, as in many areas of life, too much of a good thing can become a bad thing. When creating a program, make sure you create balance and focus on all planes of motion and functions of the muscle. What I mean by that is do not just move front to back. Sometimes, you need to incorporate lateral movements to hit areas in different ways to maintain a balanced body. Also, there are pushing and pulling exercises. If you already have rounded shoulders, chances are, you do not want to do a lot of pushing without balancing out with more pulling exercises. If you make that paper cut, it will further promote poor posture. To structure your weekly program, consider how many days a week you are going to train. Of course, there are many variations to this, but here is a simple way I would structure your weekly frequency.

When you work out two to three days per week, I suggest full-body workouts. Instead of only doing dumbbell shoulder presses and calling it shoulder day or doing squats and calling it leg day, pair them together for a full-body exercise. With the frequency you choose, you can put a day of rest in between workouts and not risk overtraining muscle groups.

On a four-day week program, I would do a two-day cycle of upper body push/pull exercises in the horizontal direction. For example, variations of row and chest presses and working the front of the legs with front squats, step-ups, and lunges. On the second day, I would do push/pull in a vertical direction. For example, variations of shoulder presses and lat pulldowns and working the back of your legs with back squats, deadlifts, and leg presses.

On a five-day week program, I would do an upper body push/pull day and then a lower body front day. Follow it with a full day of cardio and core-based activities. Then come back to an upper body push/pull day and end with legs again, specifically focusing on the back of the legs.

If you plan on working out more than five days a week, which I do not advise, then dedicate that sixth day to recovery activities like hiking, yoga, or swimming. Pick something that does not tax your body too much.

The above example is what I would do for weight loss, but with goals shifting, the workouts would change as well. Why? Because you always want to be doing that regimen that will bring your closest to your goal. You do this to maximize the return on the investment of your precious and limited time. The bottom line is that it is not just about a good sweat session. You must have a weekly and monthly plan that outlines your progressive program.

The last paper cut I want to mention is that people take advice from "specialists" that come from the "here is how I did it" approach. Well, if they are not your gender or in your age group, chances are their methods are not best for you. Here is the harsh reality you are facing. Most of these health coach gurus are in their twenties, where they can get away with improper nutrition and training and still lose weight and avoid injury. If you are no longer in your 20s, their methods may not work for you, or worse, they may hurt you in the process. Now, the advice you want to take is from coaches who have helped hundreds of people in many different demographics or from those who are in your demographic. They understand all the different ways to accomplish the same result. They apply the perfect methods for your body, and they do not cram a plan into your lifestyle. Instead, they build a plan around your lifestyle. There are no guarantees in fitness. Your body and environment are not always simple, but to get as close to a guarantee as you can, you want to take the material covered to heart.

To cap off this chapter, I want you to think about the number one factor to your success. Before considering specifics of what you do or eat, you have to approach everything with consistency first. Whether it is meal frequency or getting your butt to the gym, you need to focus on the action before outcomes. With time, you will be amazed at what you can accomplish for your health.

CHAPTER 24

Warm-Up Paper Cut

If you played sports in your early days, before starting a game or practice, you warmed up your body for activity. For some reason, as we get older, we lose that habit. We often jump into our workouts before giving our body the proper time to get ready. This paper cut impacts your ability to prepare for the session emotionally. You fail to signal to your body what muscles you want to use, and you fail to work on correcting small imbalances created from your everyday activities. By not warming up, the problems could become more significant if you do not address them before the real intensity begins. But my favorite warm-up benefit is applied to weight loss. If you warm up properly, you can increase your fat burn during a workout by about 15 percent.

I used to teach boot camp classes many years ago, and in the beginning, I struggled to retain clients and build numbers for my class. Even though I acquired new group members often, I would have low retention and, therefore, could not expand the class. I started paying attention to my body language and noticed that I was jumping into hardcore things way too soon. I was not gradually building up the workouts. When I switched to a longer and functional warm-up, suddenly, I started teaching huge classes. I saw that people were coming in tight from sitting too much, and their emotions and breathing were all over the place. Mentally, they were not prepped to push. So, I decided to incorporate more time to open their tight hips, backs, and shoulders. I created breathing exercises to keep their breath away from their chest and more focused in their diaphragm. I also gave them a bit of a pep talk to get their mind pumped up while we were getting their bodies rested. When attendance frequency picked up, I got feedback from my classes on why they felt like coming again. The answer was simple. They told me that, often, when they thought about going to the gym to see me, they would instantly associate the experience with high intensity. When feeling a bit tired or not motivated, they had no desire to come in. When I changed the format to allow for a more significant warm-up, they started to associate it with making their body feel better. They focused on getting their mind right and becoming more functional. They knew that, even if they were not in the mood, by showing up and starting with some basic warm-ups, they gradually reached a motivated state.

Throughout our lives, we do many repetitive motions that tend to put our body out of alignment and balance. Things like sitting, computer work, cellphone use, and many others, create movement patterns that were not intended as designed. These natural parts of life can lead to pain, injury, and ultimately lack of performance. Your body basically creates a memory on how it should move when it wants to accomplish a particular task. These patterns must be broken, and a warm-up is a perfect place to do that. By focusing on light and controlled movements, we signal to the system that, no, we want you to use these muscles. You accomplish this through props, angles, and the regression of a movement until it can be done with perfect control and flawless form. Often, we need to activate our glutes and our core to ensure that we do not have back pain from doing large movements with a lot of weight. We must employ more of our upper back muscles to keep our body balanced. That way, our dominant front muscles, like our chest and shoulder muscles, do not pull our joints out of alignment. This warm-up activation is important because, alternatively, you could be pushing your body hard but going in the wrong direction.

This last one is my favorite because many do warm-ups, but they do so inefficiently. Often, we bend over and touch our toes because our gym teacher had taught us that. It is not optimal and can actually weaken you prior to your lifting. Stretching is essential, and I will cover that later, but what is more critical for your body is to adjust your ability to burn fat during the workout. With weight loss goals, you always want a higher percentage of your calorie expenditure coming from your fat stores. By starting our workout with a proper warm-up, we can do exactly that. Imagine elevating your fat burn by 15 percent during your upcoming hour by doing eight minutes of something that you already do, just a little differently. Depending on your workout frequency, it can build up to an equivalent of getting an extra workout per week when it comes down to the amount of fat we can consume.

So, what should you do for a proper warm-up? As you walk into the gym, you need to dedicate about 15 minutes to warming up. This is non-negotiable. Pick the piece of cardio equipment that you enjoy the most and start with eight minutes on it, done in four two-minute segments. Start at a pace that is very easy for the first two minutes and then increase the intensity until the last two minutes. At that point you want to be moving at a pace that keeps you completely out of breath. Notice I do not say to run or sprint or dictate a specific intensity. Why? Because we are all different and are at different conditioning levels. What may be a run for me, could be a brisk jog for you and a walk to someone else. You need to gauge this with your own body.

Remember that low intensity should be somewhere where you can talk freely, and high intensity is where you are only able to say two to three words per breath. The other two rounds should be done somewhere in between those levels. Then, it is essential to take a five-minute cool down before you start your training. Even if it is strictly a cardio day, I want you to follow this format. After you complete that cardio warm-up, the next five minutes will be for stretching because now we have a great blood flow through the muscles. You can choose to use a foam roller or do some dynamic stretching. The foam roller will help work on the connective tissue that does not get much attention and is often the reason for low flexibility and mobility. Use both forms of stretching interchangeably and based on preference. After five minutes of stretching in one of those two formats, move into three minutes of light activation. Do the activation exercises in a circuit of continuous movement to maximize your time. Pick three to four movements, like glute bridges, breathing exercises, or shoulder rotations. Target the areas that you may have issues with and will be using in the upcoming workout.

This warm-up system is not the only way to do it. I am sharing what has been a staple of thousands of pounds lost by my clients. It is great because it has so many added benefits besides the 15 percent fat burn increase. I would not skip this no matter what.

CHAPTER 25

Paper Cut of Specifics

One of my clients came to me after injuring his back while lifting weights. He was a typical jock that loved sports, beer, and being a man. Due to that, he had a preconceived notion around what his fitness should look like. Most of the things he was doing in the weight room were what he had learned back in his glory days of high school football. He told me high reps and bodyweight exercises were for women. Yet, he was moving with pain every day. Waking up with a stiff back made it more challenging for him to step into the weight room for his workouts.

Over time, my client exercised less frequently, and because he maintained his eating patterns, the weight started to climb, especially around the stomach. This created more back pain and forced his body to modify his movement patterns, which made his knees hurt. He was no easy client as he thought he already knew what he wanted and how it needed to happen. In his mind, he just needed a little accountability. He told me, "I know if I just lose the weight, my back pain would go away, and my knees would stop hurting." Was he right? Yes, but only partially. If we reduce the load the body carries, it will hurt less. However, his problems had become structural because his body was imbalanced from years of heavyweight workouts without that supplemental foundational work I recommend.

So, what did we do? I had to give him a lot of what he wanted and only sprinkle in what he needed. As time passed, he began to enjoy more functional bodyweight movement as he noticed how his body felt better and better. I started seeing him come to the gym on his own and doing the things that we worked on, never touching the weights. His weight came off, he became incredibly consistent, and there were so many social improvements for him because he moved without pain. I still check in with him from time to time, and he tells me that he hardly does anything heavy. His old school workouts are around 20 percent of what he does now.

What is our lesson to take away here? Often, we are told what exercises are best for our health. Some people tell you that if you want to increase your flexibility, you need to do yoga two to three times a week. What if you hate working out with a group of people and feel self-conscious? Will it likely make you stick to that regimen? Chances are that the answer is no. Instead, look up some yoga videos and find an empty corner to stretch. You will feel better emotionally about that task and be more likely to do it for the long-term. You would be amazed how far you can get with a little consistency that comes from enjoyment. So, the lesson is that before you worry about doing the perfect exercises for your goals, first become consistent with exercising. This may take a few months, and that is perfectly fine because you are in it to win it with a marathon approach. You now understand the point of the long game.

We often subconsciously demotivate ourselves by saying that what we are doing is not good enough. You say things like, "I know I just went for a walk, but I should be running on a treadmill for an hour because that is what I put into my head." Instead of feeling good about the walk and increasing your enjoyment, you may push yourself to the treadmill too soon. This will cause you to fall off the regimen all together in a couple of weeks. Instead, tell yourself how you are not there yet and that you feel great about the little progress that you make each week.

It is so vital to start or restart your health journey by focusing on areas you enjoy and are already good at. Do more of those things and increase consistency, be it with nutrition, mindfulness, exercise, or any other components that I have discussed in this book. Stop looking at how far you have left to go and celebrate how far you have come so far. Even after day one, you already did more than you did the previous week, month, or year depending on your situation. Be grateful for the ability to change your health rather than resent how much you have allowed it to degenerate.

We already get a lot of judgment from the world as it is, we do not need to add more by judging ourselves. There will be a time where you can do the perfect exercise, nutrient intake, or stress management application, but for now, just celebrate that you have started the journey and simply remind yourself of these two words: not yet.

CONCLUSION

I want to thank you from the bottom of my heart for picking up a copy of this book, but even more importantly, for reading it all the way to the end. It is not the sexy things that Instagram influencers would push on you, like six-pack abs in 30 days, but it is the blueprint for how you can use your health as the vehicle to a thriving life.

There was a tremendous amount of information covered, and it can be overwhelming. If you are currently making a lot of these paper cuts, do not beat yourself up and try to fix everything at once. Remember that this book and the #10PercentFITTER method are based on and advocate for small yet mighty steps. I would rather you go slow, stay consistent, and build the winning momentum that helps you to move mountains. You did not get into the situation that you are in overnight, so you will not get out of it overnight, either. Yet, with consistency, you will not be able to recognize your mind, body, and spirit once they are optimized.

I encourage you to reread this book at different points in your life because different paper cuts will resonate with you more at certain times. Also, these paper cuts are not like an on and off switch but are more like a sliding scale. When you think you have optimized a particular area, you may believe that it is as good as it gets. Yet, when you improve other areas connected to it, new opportunities for improvement arise as you raise your health ceiling.

One of the best ways to ensure that you understand and maintain the information is to teach it to others. Share it with your loved ones, coworkers, and people at your gym as often as you possibly can. It will make you feel empowered and will create long-lasting habits that make it easy to live a healthy life. You will be surprised by how great it feels to be the health expert among the people around you.

Last, but most certainly not least, please share your journey to inspire others, to push the #10PercentFITTER movement, and increase world health by 10 percent. Do not be afraid to celebrate small wins on social media. Do not be afraid to show off your new clothes. Most importantly, do not be afraid to share your goals publicly to create accountability. Through this process, you will be a light for so many others that may be in the darkness. Pick up a copy of the book and send it to someone you care about because #10PercentFITTER is not just a method; it will become a worldwide movement!

www.ingramcontent.com/pod-product-compliance
Lightning Source LLC
Chambersburg PA
CBHW052134270326
41930CB00012B/2882